CALLING OF AN ANGEL

DR. GARY L. GLUM

CALLING OF AN ANGEL

SILENT WALKER
PUBLISHING
LOS ANGELES

Copyright ©1988 by Dr. Gary L. Glum
All rights reserved under International and Pan-American
Copyright conventions. Published in the United States by
Silent Walker Publishing, Los Angeles.

ISBN 0-9620364-0-4

Manufactured in the United States of America
Typography and binding design by Silent Walker Publishing

First Edition

Dedicated to

Joyce E. Thomas

There are no words to thank you.
Such power is held by few.
Such gentleness is held by only the very powerful.
To have both traits is rare.
So rare they are recognized by only a few.

On October 5, 1983, E. Bruce Hendrick, the chief of neurosurgery at the University of Toronto's Hospital for Sick Children, wrote to the Canadian Minister of Health and Welfare saying that Dr. Hendrick supported a scientific clinical trial of the cancer treatment compound known as "Essiac."

Dr. Hendrick stated that after they started on Essiac, eight of ten patients with surgically treated tumors of the central nervous system had "escaped from the conventional methods of therapy including both radiation and chemotherapy."

Dr. Hendrick wrote that he was "most impressed with the effectiveness of the treatment and its lack of side effects." He closed with this: "I feel that this method of treatment should be given serious consideration and would benefit from a scientific clinical trial."

With that letter Dr. Hendrick joined a long list of physicians dating back more than 60 years who have spoken in favor of Essiac as a cancer treatment.

Yet Essiac today remains unavailable—almost impossible to get—for nearly all cancer patients.

How could something like this happen?

INTRODUCTION

This is the story of a woman named Rene Caisse. For more than 50 years, until her death in 1978 at the age of 90, she treated thousands of cancer patients, most of them written off by doctors as terminally ill, with her own secret herbal formula. She called it Essiac—Caisse spelled backwards—and she brewed the tea herself, alone in her kitchen.

Her patients swore by her. They were devoted. Men and women who believed she cured them of cancer told their friends and families, wrote letters to doctors and politicians, swore affidavits, testified before the Canadian parliament and pleaded with Rene Caisse to supply them with more Essiac when they needed it. Some husbands and wives of patients who died wrote Rene letters thanking her profoundly for making life easier—free of pain—and longer for their loved ones. Her funeral in the village of Bracebridge, about 170 kilometers north of Toronto, was attended by hundreds of people, including former patients Rene had treated for terminal cancer as far back as the 1930s and who were still on their feet to bury her and tell their stories.

I'm convinced that Essiac works. It has potent healing—and preventive—power. It is a gift from nature. I've seen a small part of the evidence with my own eyes, and I've experienced Essiac's power as a healthful tonic in my own life. I suffered from chronic bronchitis until a few years ago when I first heard of Essiac and tried it myself. Within days my cough disappeared and it hasn't returned. I still drink the Essiac. It tastes like what it is, an herbal tea. About as plain and mild as any of the other herbal teas from around the world you can buy in any supermarket. I've never felt better. All through Canada and in parts of the United States today there are people of all ages who are absolutely convinced that Essiac saved their lives or the lives of friends and loved ones. But you can't buy it in any supermarket.

Claims have been made—since about 1925, in fact—that Essiac is an effective treatment for cancer. So the governments of North America have classified it as a "drug." The Canadian government almost legalized its use by Rene in 1939, and has gone through fits and starts ever since in deciding how to handle the situation. The policy has ranged from threatening to arrest Rene if she didn't close her clinic to promising her publicly—on the record, in the press—that she wouldn't be arrested if she would agree to keep her clinic open, thus quieting the public clamor that arose after the government threatened to shut her down.

In the last decade, the Canadian government has classified Essiac as an "experimental drug," and then an "experimental drug" that had failed to show promise, and today—as Dr. Hendrick's letter shows—the internal battles are still going on in Canada over the future of Essiac.

In the U.S., a 1978 class action suit in federal court in Detroit seeking to authorize the importation of Essiac for cancer treatment was defeated by the government. Other than that, the U.S. government hasn't faced much pressure about Essiac. There are probably high level officials in the U.S. Food and Drug Administration—and the National Cancer Institute—who make life and death decisions about cancer drugs who could honestly say they've never heard of Essiac. I hope they'll take the time to read this book.

I don't claim that Essiac is a miraculous panacea, capable of curing all cancers in all people, nor do I believe that. Rene Caisse didn't even believe that. She didn't claim Essiac as a "cure for cancer." Her former patients were the ones who put forward that claim, strenuously and over many decades. What Rene maintained was that Essiac caused regression in some cancerous tumors, the total destruction of others, prolonged life in most cases and—in virtually every case—significantly diminished the pain and suffering of cancer patients.

If the testimonials of Rene's former patients, including those sworn under oath, have any credibility at all—and when I present them, I think you'll agree they do—then Essiac's powers as a pain reliever in cancer patients are nothing short of phenomenal. In sixty years of personal accounts, the easing of agony and an increased sense of well-being—often to the point of getting through the day without narcotics—is one of the predominant themes. You hear it over and over again, and always told with a deep sense of gratitude.

Rene fought almost her whole adult life against overwhelming odds and under incredible pressures, some of them self-imposed, to establish those simple facts as accepted wisdom. She never gave up her fight. But for one woman many years ago to persuade the medical and legal institutions of North America that a natural treatment for cancer—based on herbs that grow wild— might make more sense than the accepted means of surgery, radiation and chemotherapy...she might as well have been telling them in an earlier century that the earth is round.

Remember: Rene was fighting cancer with a natural treatment in an era when the conventional wisdom of the medical establishment denied even that diet might be a factor in causing cancer. It's hard to believe, knowing what we know now—and what has become the conventional wisdom—but for generations those doctors who preached dietary causes of cancer were dismissed by most physicians as quacks. So what was the medical establishment to make of this woman—who wasn't even a licensed doctor—who preached that a cancer treatment was to be found in plants that grow wild?

My goal in this book is simple: I want to tell the story of this ordinary woman's extraordinary life and share the knowledge of Essiac so that people can make their own informed decisions about what its future should be. I don't pretend to have all the answers about how and why Essiac works, or the final scientific proof that it does. There are large gaps, as I'll explain, in my own knowledge of this story. Much of it remains a mystery to me, raising deeply intriguing questions which I would love to see answered.

But I do know that there is already enough evidence that Essiac has benefited cancer patients in the last 60 years to warrant those controlled clinical studies that some physicians—such as Dr. Hendrick—have advocated for decades.

The risk to the public would certainly appear to be minimal. There seems to be universal agreement among the doctors and scientists who have done investigations of Essiac—and the patients who have used it—that Essiac is non-toxic and without harmful side effects. Rene Caisse drank it every day for half a century and some of her family and close friends always made sure they had their daily cup. Not even Rene Caisse's worst enemies ever put forward the argument that people were hurt by drinking the tea.

This non-toxic nature of Essiac is an important consideration in making it a treatment worthy of serious investigation. Many of the conventionally accepted chemotherapy drugs actually come with toxic warning labels. One of the commonly administered cancer drugs is the chemical Fluorouracil (5 FU). Note this warning on the manufacturer's brochure: "Precautions: Fluorouracil is a highly toxic drug with a narrow margin of safety. Therefore, patients should be carefully supervised since therapeutic response is unlikely to occur without some evidence of toxicity....Severe hematological toxicity, gastrointestinal hemorrhage and even death may result from the fluorouracil despite meticulous selection of patients and careful adjustment of dosage."

As if that weren't bad enough, the officially accepted "experimental drugs," on which the government and the drug companies lavish huge sums of developmental funds, can be even worse. According to a 1981 Washington Post story, a major American drug company spent significant amounts of money and years of research on a weed from India they hoped would have a beneficial effect on certain forms of leukemia—even though it was known in advance that the weed caused severe liver damage in livestock. And sure enough, when the weed was synthesized into a chemical and given to cancer patients, there were reports that it was helping some people—and killing others.

But there was nothing unusual in that. "We knew from the beginning that this caused toxicity in animals," the Post quoted a U.S. Food and Drug Administration official as saying. "Almost all investigational cancer drugs are highly toxic." As you read this story and wonder—as I did many, many times while I was researching it—if an herbal compound developed by one woman could possibly—even possibly—be safer and more effective than the best of what medical science is already bringing us, please

keep this quote in mind from that same 1981 series of Washington *Post* articles:

"Over the last decade, more than 150 experimental drugs have been given to tens of thousands of cancer patients under the sponsorship of the US Federal Government's National Cancer Institute. Many of these drugs have come from a list of highly toxic industrial chemicals, including pesticides, herbicides and dyes....While all anti-cancer drugs can cause side effects among some of those who take them, the experimental drugs—along with leading to hundreds of deaths—have elicited a nightmarish list of serious adverse reactions, including kidney failure, liver failure, heart failure, respiratory distress, destruction of bone marrow so the body can no longer make blood, brain damage, paralysis, seizure, coma and visual hallucinations.

"So little is known about many of these chemicals that doctors have found these ironic results: In some cases the experimental drug actually stimulated tumor growth rather than stopped the cancer—and in other tests, doctors and researchers found that the experimental drug itself caused cancer."

Rene Caisse wouldn't have been surprised to read that. Her own feelings about the use of these toxic drugs, after a lifetime spent fighting cancer, were blunt and nasty: "Chemotherapy should be a criminal offense," she told one reporter.

Though the medical establishment has not yet recognized Rene Caisse's herbal treatment for cancer as legitimate, there is more than ample precedent for the approach she was taking. According to a 1987 NOVA documentary on "The Hidden Power of Plants," aired on the Public Broadcasting System: "Indeed, the history of medicine has been largely the story of plants and the potent chemicals they produce. Around the world, traditional healers, using plant medications, provide health care to eighty percent of the human population—over four billion people."

Since the 1950s doctors have been using an alkaloid called vincristine—which comes from an evergreen plant known as the periwinkle—in the treatment of childhood leukemia and other cancers. Digitalis, which comes from the leaves of the foxglove plant, is an important heart medication. According to the NOVA documentary, "Over 25 percent of the drugs prescribed in the U.S. still contain plant materials as their principal active ingredients."

Throughout history there are countless examples of people discovering the healing properties of nature before science could understand them—or even believe that they existed. South American Indians treated fevers, especially malarial fevers, with an herbal tea made from cinchona bark. Scientists eventually discovered that cinchona bark is nature's source of quinine.

Science didn't discover that Vitamin C prevented scurvy. English sailors discovered that without even knowing it. All they knew was that they'd better take some citrus fruits—lemons, limes—along with them on long ocean voyages. That's why the English came to be called "limeys." Science didn't even discover Vitamin C until 1932.

For centuries, American Indians treated various aches and pains with an herbal tea made from white willow bark. It must have seemed terribly primitive to the doctors who first heard of it. They were trusting their science; the Indians were trusting nature. But eventually science caught up. Today, synthesized and refined white willow bark is the basis for what we call aspirin.

Always, in all cultures, there was what might be called "living proof" of the medicinal value of plants long before there was scientific proof—and acceptance. Living proof, of course, is not acceptable to the scientific community. Not even the testimony of ordinary individuals, sworn to oath, meets the rigorous standards of scientific proof. But no matter what happens in the scientific world, living proof will be what passes from person to person and prevents Essiac from dying out altogether in the modern world.

Rene Caisse's files are filled with letters from people all over North America testifying to life-saving experiences with Essiac. Almost 400 people showed up at the Canadian Cancer Commission hearings in 1939 prepared to be sworn to oath and state that Essiac saved their lives.

Today, all over Canada and in parts of the U.S., there are thousands of people who may not know the first thing about scientific proof, but who know that Essiac benefited or even saved them or someone they love. For science to deny that there is a cause and effect relationship between Essiac and the relief of pain and the regression of cancerous tumors is almost like saying, well, we can see all those great huge billowing clouds of smoke, but we haven't been able to determine with certainty that there is a fire.

While most Americans have never heard of Essiac, the controversy it inspires has raged in Canada since the 1920s, every few years in the public glare of the press, and frequently involving the highest medical, legal and political circles in Canada. But always that controversy centered on this one woman who lived, most of the time, in the tiny village of Bracebridge, Ontario, population 9,000 or so.

Rene Caisse was an unlikely public figure. She was a skilled nurse who didn't crave attention or money. "I never had $100 I could call my own," she used to laugh with her friends. She didn't charge a fee for her services. She accepted only voluntary contributions—in the form of fruits, vegetables or eggs, as often as not—from those who could afford to offer them, and she didn't turn away people who couldn't make any payment at all.

One man, Ted Hale, was so grateful watching his wife recover from cancer using Essiac that he slipped a $50 bill under a book on a shelf when he came to pick up another bottle from Rene. The next time he arrived at her front door, he says, she grabbed him by his shirt collar, pulled him inside and gave him a piece of her mind. How dare he leave her that much money? She didn't like it one bit. He apologized and asked her if she would accept it as his way of donating for the next people who needed her Essiac and couldn't afford to leave anything at all. She finally relented on those grounds and kept the money, but Ted Hale still laughs at his own embarrassment when he tells the story ten years later.

Rene Caisse lived her whole life in modest circumstances while rejecting offers of vast sums of money to reveal her formula. She refused to reveal her formula to people who wanted to help her; she refused to reveal her formula to powerful institutions that demanded it before they would consider legitimizing Essiac. What Rene Caisse wanted was to heal the ill and guarantee the legalization of Essiac for all, yet her intransigent refusal to budge from secrecy about the formula cost her—and us—dearly.

She refused to reveal the formula to the Canadian government, the Memorial Sloan-Kettering Cancer Center in New York—the world's largest private cancer research center—and the National Cancer Institute, just to name some of the institutions that wanted the formula at one time or another. She wouldn't give them the formula until they would admit that Essiac had merit as a treatment for cancer. They refused to admit any merit until she gave them the formula.

There were legitimate arguments made on both sides. Rene was fearful that the medical establishment would either exploit Essiac, charging exorbitant prices to make a fortune and placing it beyond the means of the poor, or discredit it and bury it. The doctors and politicians argued that they couldn't very well accept the legitimacy of a cancer treatment if they didn't even know what was in it. The result was a tragic standoff.

We have lost decades of precious research. With hindsight, it can be argued that Rene Caisse should have given the formula to anyone, anywhere, at any time, who wanted to have it for any reason, on the grounds that the more people who have it, the better chance that the truth will out. That certainly will be the position taken in this book.

I am going to release to the public, for the first time, the formula and the procedure for preparing Essiac. I will explain in detail at the end of this book how I will do that, and how anyone who wants that information may have it.

I believe that information should be in the hands of the public. People should have the right to make their own decisions about whether or not they will drink the Essiac tea. People can make it themselves, if they wish, just the way Rene did. The herbs are available for less than $50 from any major herbal distributor in America. There is no mystery about the preparation. It must be done carefully and accurately—as I will explain—but it finally comes down to: Put in so much of this herb, so much of that herb, brew it and drink the tea.

The herbs themselves grow in many regions. Rene used to say that enough of the herbs grow in Ontario to supply the whole world. But in revealing the formula, I share one of Rene's deep fears that played an important role in her refusal to release the formula until after the governing bodies of medicine and law would admit that it had merit: Namely, that once the herbs are publicly identified, these inexpensive and widely available plants will be placed on the federal "controlled substances" roster—like some dangerous drug—and suddenly become very difficult—and illegal—to acquire.

But there's nothing I can do about that. As always, those decisions are up to the governments. But my decision is to tell the story of how I came into possession of the formula, place it before the public and let people make up their own minds about what they want to do with it. At least once the formula is in the public domain, the old argument that was used for so long against Rene—we can't do proper scientific studies until we know the formula—will no longer have any validity at all. Sloan-Kettering, for instance, was telling Rene Caisse at least as late as 1975 that they would perform more clinical studies on Essiac, if only they had the formula. Well, now they'll have it. And so will anyone who wants it.

Rene Caisse was a sweet woman who gave her best and saw the worst. She was surrounded most of her life with the pain and suffering of others. She lived under siege much of the time, with a legion of supporters who saw her as a saint and powerful enemies who wanted her arrested for practicing medicine without a license. She became so fearful and paranoid about arrest that she sometimes had to turn away dying people who were pleading with her to help them. But more often, she found ways to help the people who came to her, even total strangers who had nothing to offer her. She said once about her situation: "I was always just one jump ahead of a policeman. We were right across the street from the town jail and the keeper used to joke that he was saving a cell for me."

The blessing of Essiac brought a curse for Rene Caisse: Her life was never her own.

CHAPTER
ONE

I n 1922, Rene Caisse was a 33-year-old surgical nurse in Haileybury, Ontario. The physicians and surgeons she assisted, by all accounts, held her in high esteem. She had established an excellent reputation as a nurse.

Her family was prominent in the Bracebridge area. Her parents were among the local pioneers who had first settled there in the 1870s when that remote part of Canada was opened up by the lumber and fur trapping industries.

Rene's father ran the local barber shop and was active in civic affairs; her mother was active in church affairs. They raised their 12 children to be good Catholics, and Rene—the 8th of 12— remained faithful to the church all her life.

The old, fading photographs of the Caisses and their 12 children posed for portraits show a handsome, well-dressed family. The few photographs that survive of Rene as a young woman in her nursing uniform show her to be trim and strikingly beautiful, dark haired with shining eyes.

Those photographs come as a surprise even to people who knew her in the years after she discovered Essiac. At some point early on in those years, she let herself go physically and became terribly overweight, well over 200 pounds, and she stayed that way for the rest of her life. But when she was young, Rene Caisse was a real beauty.

One day in 1922, Rene was caring for an old woman who had just come out of surgery. The woman's right breast was badly scarred. Rene asked the woman what had happened to her. As Rene later described the scene, many times over many years and always the same way, the woman told Rene that she had come from England 30 years earlier to join her husband, who was prospecting in northern Ontario. Not long after she arrived in Canada, her right breast had become sore and swollen and painful. An old Indian medicine man at the mining camp had told her that she had cancer and he could cure it with an Indian herbal remedy. He would be happy to give it to her.

But instead her husband had taken her to doctors in Toronto. The doctors told her that she was suffering from advanced cancer, and the breast would have to be removed at once. She didn't want the surgery. One of her friends had recently died from the same operation, and they couldn't afford the surgery, anyway, so she decided she'd take her chances with the old Indian.

When they got back to the mining camp, the Indian gave the woman an herbal tea to drink and told her the ingredients and how to prepare it so that she could make her own when she needed more. She drank the tea every day for some time and gradually her tumors diminished in size, then disappeared. Her breast was left scarred, but more than 20 years later, she was still free of cancer. She was nearly 80 when she told Rene her story.

"I was much interested," Rene said years later, "and wrote down the names of the herbs she had used. I knew that doctors threw up their hands when cancer was discovered in a patient; it was the same as a death sentence, just about. I decided that if I should ever develop cancer, I would use this herb tea.

"About a year later I was visiting an aged, retired doctor whom I knew well. We were walking slowly about his garden when he took his cane and lifted a weed. 'Nurse Caisse,' he told me, 'if people would use this weed there would be little or no cancer in the world.'

"He told me the name of the plant. It was one of the herbs my patient had named as an ingredient of the medicine man's tea."

Rene always made it clear that she didn't immediately do anything with the information. She had no way of knowing whether to believe it, and she was busy with her nursing, so she just filed it away in case she might ever need it in the future.

The future came suddenly. A few months after she strolled in the garden with the doctor, Rene got word that her mother's only sister had been operated on in Brockville, Ontario. She had cancer of the stomach with a liver involvement. She was given six months to live—at most.

Rene: "I hastened to her and talked to her doctor. He was Dr. R.O. Fisher of Toronto, whom I knew well for I'd nursed patients for him many times. I told him about the herb tea and asked his permission to try it under his observation, since there apparently was nothing more medical science could do for my aunt. He consented quickly."

Thinking she had nothing to lose, Rene gathered the herbs and brewed the tea. According to Rene's account, her aunt drank the tea for two months, gradually got stronger and eventually recovered. (And lived for another 21 years.) Rene had her first convert in the medical community: Dr. R. O. Fisher. "Dr. Fisher was so impressed that he asked me to use my treatment on some of his other hopeless cancer cases," Rene said years later.

Over the next decade, it became common knowledge that Rene and Dr. Fisher were, in fact, treating patients. Those patients showed enough improvement to convince Dr. Fisher that Rene

Caisse was on to an important discovery. He became one of her strongest advocates, and, according to Rene, the person who suggested to her that they could achieve even more dramatic results if she would inject the substance hypodermically.

Rene later recalled her first injection of a human patient. A man from Lyons, New York, a patient of Dr. Fisher's, had cancer of the throat and tongue. "Dr. Fisher wanted me to inject Essiac into the tongue. Well, I was nearly scared to death. And there was a violent reaction. The patient developed a severe chill; his tongue swelled so badly the doctor had to press it down with a spatula to let him breathe. That lasted about 20 minutes. Then the swelling went down, the chill subsided, and the patient was all right. The cancer stopped growing, the patient went home, and he lived quite comfortably for almost four years."

But it was obvious to Rene that she needed to learn a lot more about the herbs before she injected any more patients. At the same time, she still had to earn a living, so she kept her nursing job and put in long days at the hospital. Her nights and weekends she spent in her mother's basement in Toronto, which she had converted into a laboratory, injecting different combinations of the herbs into mice that had been inoculated with human cancers.

Rene concluded that one of the herbs reduced the growth of the tumors; the other herbs worked as blood purifiers, cleansing the system of destroyed tissue and infections sloughed off by the malignancies. "I found that the ingredients which stopped the malignancy growth could be given by intramuscular injection in the forearm to destroy the mass of malignant cells, and giving the medicine orally to purify the blood, I got quicker results than when the medicine was all given orally."

Meanwhile, word was spreading that this nurse was having success in treating cancer patients with her herbal formula. Some of Dr. Fisher's colleagues began asking Rene to treat their hopeless cases. One of those patients was an 80-year-old man whose face was so ravaged by cancer that his doctors said he couldn't live more than ten days.

Rene: "'We will not expect a miracle,' they told me. 'But if your treatment can help this man in this stage of cancer, we will know that you have discovered something the whole world needs desperately.' My treatment stopped the bleeding in less than 24 hours. The man's face healed. He lived for six months, with very little discomfort."

In 1926, nine licensed Canadian physicians, who had seen the results of Rene's work, took the unusual and dramatic step of petitioning Canada's Department of Health and Welfare to allow Rene to conduct large-scale tests of Essiac. The petition read:

We, the undersigned, believe that the 'Treatment for Cancer' given by Nurse R.M. Caisse can do no harm and that it relieves pain, will reduce the enlargement and will prolong life in hopeless cases.

To the best of our knowledge, she has not been given a case to treat until everything in Medical and Surgical Science had been tried without effect, and even then, she was able to show remarkably beneficial results, on these cases, at that late stage.

We would be interested to see her given an opportunity to prove her work in a large way.

To the best of our knowledge she has treated all cases free of any charge and has been carrying on this work over the period of the past two years.

Signed,
R.O. Fisher, R.C.P.,M.R.C.S.
J.X. Robert, M.B.

R.A. Blye, M.B.

C.E. Becker, M.D.C.M.

E.F. Hoidge, M.B.,L.R.C.P.,M.R.C.S.

J.A. McInnis, M.D.

Chas. H. Hair, M.D.C.M.

A. Moore, M.D.C.M.

W.F. Williams, M.D.

Rene Caisse was naive enough to believe that her work would now be recognized and advanced through official channels. In her own description, she was "joyful beyond words at this expression of confidence by such outstanding doctors regarding the benefits derived from my treatment."

But her joy was short-lived. The petition backfired. It became the opening gun in the war over Essiac. The government wasted no time pouncing on this nurse who was practicing medicine. The Department of Health and Welfare immediately dispatched two of their doctors to investigate Rene. Carrying official papers that authorized them to have her arrested—or restrained from practicing without a license—they showed up without warning at her front door.

Rene was badly shaken, but she explained to them that she was only treating patients who had been given up—abandoned—by their physicians as terminally ill, and she was accepting only voluntary contributions. She made no charge for her services. She showed them her papers, her reports, her letters from physicians. They listened to what she had to say and decided to back off. They told her they were not going to have her arrested, nor were they going to order her to stop doing what she'd been doing.

Rene won that battle, but the war was on. For the next fifteen years she lived under siege. As the word of her cancer treatment spread—in largest part by former patients and their friends and families, as well as hundreds of newspaper articles all over Canada—Rene treated dozens, and later hundreds, of patients a month while the doctors and officials who wanted her arrested fought—in parliament, in the press, in the government bureaucracy—with the doctors and officials who believed in her and wanted her left alone to do her work.

One of the two doctors first sent by the Department of Health and Welfare in 1926 to investigate and perhaps arrest Rene was Dr. W.C. Arnold. He was so impressed with what he saw that he made arrangements for her to carry on her experiments with mice at the Christie Street Hospital in Toronto, under the supervision of two of the hospital's physicians. (Dr. Arnold, who later became chief physician of the Canadian Pension Board, corresponded with Rene for the next 15 years, writing her long letters of encouragement, giving her advice in her political battles, helping her round up support and—always—trying to persuade her to release the formula to him.)

Looking back many years later on her days in the Christie Street Hospital laboratory, Rene said: "Those mice were inoculated with Rous Sarcoma. I kept them alive 52 days—which was longer than anyone else had been able to do."

Physicians continued to send cancer patients to Rene. One of the doctors who signed the petition in 1926 went even further in 1929. He put into writing at great length and in painful detail exactly what happened with one of the cancer patients he referred to Rene Caisse.

The two-page, single-spaced letter, dated March 22, 1929, and signed by Dr. J.A. McInnis, tells the story of a 55-year-old woman identified only as Mrs. DeCarle. She first visited him, he wrote, in late 1928. She was suffering severe abdominal pains. He examined her and found a tumor in her upper abdomen.

"This tumor was hard and nodular to the touch. There was also another mass which could be distinctly palpated in the region of the uterus."

Dr. McInnis then wrote: "From the history of her case, symptoms and physical examination, I had no hesitation in arriving at a diagnosis of carcinoma." Later he was informed by Mrs. DeCarle's family that she had been under the care of two specialists in Brockville who believed that the condition was malignant and that Mrs. DeCarle had only several months to live.

"As this case was inoperable," Dr. McInnis stated, "any treatment given her could only be of a palliative nature and we began to administer Miss Caisse's treatment for cancer on December 3rd. The medicine was in liquid form and given orally, twice daily. After the first ten days treatment, quite an improvement was observed, both in the patient's condition generally and in connection with the two tumors I have described, in regard to size and consistency. The abdomen was less rigid, her appetite was improved and the discomfort and pain after eating was considerably lessened."

In his examinations of Mrs. DeCarle over the next several weeks, Dr. McInnis stated, he found that the tumors in her abdomen and her pelvis were becoming smaller, and the nodular condition of the growths was disappearing. "In addition, the general health and condition of the patient improved wonderfully. Each week she felt better and was able to remain up for the greater part of the day, could eat well, pain and discomfort had disappeared and she began occupying herself with house work, besides which, she was gaining in weight."

Mrs. DeCarle was treated until March lst, "when her general condition of health appeared normal. The growth in the upper abdomen reduced, at least, by more than two thirds of its former size, the nodular condition entirely disappeared, and what remained would appear to be only adhesions from rolled up omentum. The tumor in the pelvis was scarcely palpable at all."

Dr. McInnis then described Mrs. DeCarle as looking "in normal health." She had told him she was feeling as well as she ever did, and she had gained 20 pounds. "Altogether, I would say that the treatment has brought about a remarkable transformation. Whether the results so far obtained from Miss Caisse's treatment will be permanent, remains to be seen. I am of the opinion that these results are conclusive."

Dr. McInnis noted that no X-ray had been taken before the treatment was begun, and no X-ray had been taken since the end of the treatment. But: "At the time the gastric series were made, films indicated the presence of the two masses I have described and were strongly indicative of carcinoma."

He concluded: "I desire to state that the results of Miss Caisse's treatment have been decidedly remarkable and I have no hesitation in making the statement that this treatment has reduced the growths to a minimum, has entirely relieved pain and has apparently restored the patient to normal health."

Even physicians whose skepticism initially bordered on hostility were being won over by what they saw. A typical example is Dr. J. Masson Smith of Beaverton, Ontario. On February 23, 1932, he addressed a curt "Dear Madam" letter to Rene informing her, in the briefest possible terms, that Mr. F. Maxwell appeared to have "malignant disease in his Pancreas."

Dr. Smith listed the symptoms—loss of appetite, loss of 20 pounds, extreme weakness—and said that Mr. Maxwell "wishes to undertake your treatment." The doctor reluctantly offered no objections.

Five weeks later, on March 30, 1932, Dr. Smith wrote a second letter to Rene. This time he couldn't have been friendlier—and it was obvious how impressed he was. "Mr. F. Maxwell came to my office Sunday last," Dr. Smith wrote. "Frankly, I was delighted to see such a marked improvement in his general health.

"He has gained seven and a half pounds. His hemoglobin estimated ninety percent. He moves with a great deal more vigor and mentally he is very much brighter and alert.

"I would be interested to know something more definite of your treatment. With what particular conditions do you use it and what do you claim for it? Over what period of time do you believe it should be used? I will watch Mr. Maxwell's progress with a great deal of interest."

(Mr. Maxwell's progress, as it turned out, was very good. In Rene Caisse's files is a letter from him, dated five years later, in which he says his brother is now sick and asks if Rene would please treat him. "He knows just as much and more than I do what you did for me," Mr. Maxwell wrote in 1937.)

With results like that, Rene's life was going through a complete upheaval. As many as 30 patients a day were showing up at her apartment for treatment. She decided she had to give up her nursing job to be able to devote full-time to her patients, and since she wasn't allowed to charge for her services, she was now dependent upon whatever voluntary contributions came her way.

The neighbors in her apartment building in Toronto objected to the constant stream of people into and out of Rene's apartment at all hours, so she was forced to move to Peterborough, east of Toronto. But she used to joke with friends that she would have had to move sooner or later anyway, because once she quit nursing to treat patients she couldn't afford the rent in Toronto.

Shortly after she moved to Peterborough, a health officer showed up at her door one morning at 8 a.m., saying that he had a warrant to arrest her for malpractice. As upset as she was, Rene calmly sat the official down, told him her whole story, showed him what she was doing and won him over.

Instead of arresting her, he returned to his boss, Dr. R.J. Noble, registrar of the Canadian College of Physicians and Surgeons, to explain the situation to him. Once again, Rene had talked her way out of the threat of a jail cell.

But she was frantic. This was already the second time she'd come within an unsympathetic ear of being arrested. So she organized her own counterattack. She took five friendly doctors and 12 of her patients to the office of the Minister of Health, Dr. Robb.

Dr. Robb heard them out and promised Rene that she wouldn't be arrested—for the time being—if she continued to accept only patients who had a written diagnosis of cancer from their doctors—and if she made no charge. That was fine with Rene. "The look of gratitude I saw in my patients' eyes when relief from pain was accomplished," she wrote years later, "and the hope and cheerfulness that returned when they saw their malignancies reducing was pay enough for all my efforts."

In 1932, the Toronto *Star* published the first major newspaper article about Rene Caisse and Essiac. The headline read: "Bracebridge Girl Makes Notable Discovery Against Cancer."

The story was now out in front of the public. Rene was 44 years old, badly overweight, under heavy stress carrying her patient load, and on her feet all day and half the night in the kitchen of her apartment cooking up Essiac.

Now she was going to be facing the additional pressures of becoming a sought after public figure and the center of a major political battle in the Canadian parliament. The battle would build in Canada for the rest of the 1930s, and what Rene went through would have destroyed someone with less determination and stamina.

But it didn't destroy Rene. In fact, she forced a national government to question the most cherished assumptions of its own legal

and medical bureaucracies. She came very close to winning official acceptance and recognition for her treatment of cancer
patients with Essiac.

CHAPTER
TWO

Almost immediately after the Toronto *Star* newspaper article, Rene was deluged with people who needed her help or wanted to do business with her. A Toronto businessman named Ernest H. Ashley had a contract drawn up that offered Rene her own clinic, $20,000 within the first year of signing, an annual salary of $2,000, and $100,000 in operating capital and stock in the corporation to be formed—if she would "assign and set over all her right, title and interest in the said formula above referred to."

For a woman who used to laugh that she never had $100 she could call her own, the offer must have been tempting, at least for a moment. Those were big dollar figures in 1932. But Rene turned him down, stuck the unsigned contract in her files and left it there to gather dust.

As Rene treated an increasing number of patients, the word about her work continued to be positive, even in some official circles. On June 17, 1933, she received a letter on official stationery from the Deputy Minister of Hospitals for Ontario. He wrote: "Through a friend of mine here I have learned of your wonderful treatment for cancer, and I should greatly appreciate a letter setting forth briefly the nature of your treatment. Please state how long you have been using this treatment, approximately how many cases you have treated and with what results, and whether you have any testimonials or press clippings endorsing your work. If you have copies of the latter I should be glad to receive them and will return same as soon as possible. This letter is purely personal, and not official, so please feel free to write me fully."

About that same time, one of the most prominent doctors in the Bracebridge area, Dr. A.F. Bastedo, agreed to let Rene treat one of his patients who was considered to be terminally ill with bowel cancer. When the patient recovered, Dr. Bastedo persuaded the Town Council of Bracebridge to turn over to Rene—for $1.00 a month rent—the British Lion Hotel for her use as a "cancer clinic," if she would come back to her home town to practice.

The British Lion Hotel, on one of the main streets in town, within walking distance of the Municipal Building and directly across the street from the jail, had been repossessed by the village for back taxes. In 1935, Rene opened the doors.

Rene: "The Mayor and Council were very enthusiastic and with their aid and the aid of friends, relatives and patients, I furnished an office, dispensary, reception room and five treatment rooms. Here I worked for almost eight years with a large 'CANCER CLINIC' sign on the door. Doctors sent or brought their patients to me. Doctors from many parts of the United States came to watch me treat, to examine patients and observe results. Patients came from far in ambulances, but after having a few treatments, were able to walk into the clinic by themselves. They came from far and near. Here, for almost eight years, I treated thousands of patients."

Rene's account is true. The older people in the Bracebridge area still have vivid memories of Nurse Caisse and her clinic, and all the patients coming from far and near. They still talk about friends or neighbors or aunts or uncles or parents who were saved or at least helped and relieved of pain by Nurse Caisse. They speak of her with great fondness and respect—even reverence, in many cases.

One local woman now in her 60s remembers when she was 12 years old watching Nurse Caisse in her white uniform chasing the woman's parents down the street. Her father had stomach cancer, and he'd left too much money behind after his treatment. Nurse Caisse's green eyes were flashing. She said, "Don't you ever dare do that to me again." She made him take his money back.

To this day the woman still remembers her mother and father joyfully dancing together because the treatments by Nurse Caisse had taken his pain away.

Based on contemporary newspaper accounts and their own interviews with eyewitnesses, *Homemaker's*, a Canadian national magazine, later described the scene in the 1930s: "Dominion Street took on an atmosphere reminiscent of the famous Shrine of Lourdes, as hopeful pilgrims sought a new lease on life. Cars were parked solidly along its shoulders. People from all walks of life waited patiently to enter the red brick building. Some were carried. Others were pushed gently up the steps, while the rest managed on their own. Occasionally, an ambulance would shriek its arrival as it double-parked. Rene would be seen coming quickly down to it to treat a stretcher case. Always with a doctor standing by, she injected scores of patients every day."

About the time Rene opened the clinic, her 72-year-old mother was diagnosed with inoperable cancer of the liver. Four local doctors said she was too weak for surgery. But Rene called in one of Ontario's top specialists, Dr. Roscoe Graham. He confirmed the diagnosis and, in Rene's account, said: "Her liver is a nodular mass."

One of the local doctors who didn't approve of Rene's work said to her, sarcastically: "Why don't *you* do something?"

Rene replied: "I'm certainly going to try, Doctor." She asked Dr. Graham, "How long does she have to live?" Dr. Graham said he thought it was only a matter of days. According to Rene, she didn't even tell her mother she had cancer. Instead, Rene gave her daily injections of Essiac, saying it was a tonic prescribed by her doctor.

Many years later Rene reminisced: "To make a long story short, my mother completely recovered. She passed away quietly after her 90th birthday—without pain, just a tired heart. This repaid me for all of my work—giving my mother 18 years of life she would not have had without Essiac. It made up for a great deal of the persecution I have endured at the hands of the medical people."

With a nurse now openly treating large numbers of cancer patients, in her own "cancer clinic," subsidized partly by the town of Bracebridge, the political battle started to heat up. On September 14, 1935, the Ontario Minister of Health, Dr. J.A. Faulkner, wrote to Rene saying that if she expected the government to take measures to see that her remedy be put into use for all cancer patients in the Province of Ontario, she would have to turn over her formula.

"It is necessary that a full statement be submitted," he wrote, "indicating the exact nature of the materials suggested for use, the manner in which they are to be used including dosage and the experience which has attended their use, with such detailed reports on pathological diagnosis, treatment and present condition of patients as exist."

Eleven days later, Faulkner wrote to Rene again. He said that he had "chosen an outstanding scientist to investigate your treatment. If you will submit the information desired it will be referred to him for investigation and report."

Rene wasn't about to turn over the formula. She was wide open about her work; she welcomed physicians who wanted to visit her clinic and investigate for themselves what she was doing. She wanted doctors to examine her patients, talk to them, and look at the records. But until the medical profession gave official acknowledgement that Essiac had merit, Rene was determined that the formula itself would remain secret.

Meanwhile, public pressure was building in support of Rene. In a remarkable display of grassroots political action, the local residents of the Bracebridge area rounded up thousands of signatures on petitions demanding government backing for her work.

The petitions were presented to Dr. Faulkner. He also received another petition with only nine signatures—but they were all physicians, including seven who hadn't signed the original petition back in 1926. This brought to 16 the number of licensed physicians who had staked their reputations on an endorsement of Rene and Essiac.

By 1936, the Canadian press was paying close attention to the story. Articles—and letters to the editor—began to appear with some regularity throughout Ontario. There were many accounts written by people who said they had received Nurse Caisse's treatments and had been cured of cancer.

This was really the beginning of the notion that Rene Caisse was preaching that she could cure all cancer. She wasn't. She was saying that Essiac caused regression in tumors, prolonged life, relieved pain and—in the right circumstances with patients whose organs weren't already destroyed—could cure cancer. But the heartfelt tributes from grateful patients tended to simplify the message. As far as they were concerned, she cured cancer and that was all there was to it.

Typical of the letters to the editor was one signed by Herbert Rawson and published in the spring of 1936.

Rawson said that he was a middle aged man who had been getting sicker and sicker and seeing various doctors, to no avail. Finally an X-ray showed cancer. The doctors advised an operation. "I had seen so many others that have had operations that I just refused," Mr. Rawson wrote. "They sent me to Miss Caisse. That was a year ago on the 20th of April. About three weeks ago two of the best doctors examined me well and to my great joy, they told me I was a free man from that dreaded disease, cancer. These were their words: 'You will never know what you owe that girl.' So I can say that I feel in the best of health and have gained weight. No doubt Miss Caisse will be surprised to see this letter. I would sincerely ask everyone who can to help her in this great work."

Rene's results continued to impress others. One of her patients shortly after she opened her clinic was a man named John Tynan. A few years later, Tynan would testify under oath before a Canadian parliamentary commission investigating Essiac that he had been diagnosed by four different doctors as having cancer of the rectum and been given, in their estimate, about three weeks to live. "I went to the operating room again," Tynan testified, "and they didn't do anything because they couldn't, and they put me to bed and they said, you may have a few days in bed and then you may as well go home."

Tynan testified that when he left the hospital he went to Rene's clinic and took the first of 27 regular treatments. Within 24 hours, he began to feel relief. Within four days, he felt "a wonderful change," and after the first few treatments he was able to drive himself to the clinic. Four years after the treatments, he had gained 39 pounds and felt in good health.

One of the people who was familiar with the Tynan case was Dr. W.C. Arnold, the physician who had first been sent by the Minister of Health to arrest Rene. What he saw must have made a deep impression on him because buried in Rene's files is a long, handwritten letter to her from Dr. Arnold, dated February 5, 1936. In it, he discusses the pressures upon her to release the formula, urges her to let him begin testing Essiac, and then he says: "If I can get one case to respond as John Tynan did, I'll throw in with you 100% and drop everything else."

By now, the local politicians were getting involved. The mayor of Bracebridge, Wilburt Richards, visited the office of Dr. Faulkner, the Minister of Health, with a group of prominent citizens and a petition with 2,700 signatures asking that the government accept and officially authorize Rene's treatment of patients.

Whatever Dr. Faulkner actually promised them, his actions following the meeting were not enough to satisfy Rene. On May 3, 1936, she wrote to Dr. Faulkner: "You promised the deputation who waited on you and made presentation of a petition signed by 2,700 people on my behalf that you would allow me to demonstrate my treatment before doctors, of your choosing, on patients, of their choosing. This you have failed to do. You simply wrote and asked me to send the formula.

"I should think the public Health Department would be back of anyone who would try to help suffering humanity. Instead of this, I find you putting every obstacle in my way."

Rene offered this challenge to the Minister of Health: Let her send some of her patients—and their case histories, X-ray plates, and so on—for examination by doctors. "And then if you are not satisfied, I will give up this work. I could not be more reasonable than that, could I?"

The political pressure on Rene's behalf appeared to be paying off. On July 10, 1936, a headline in the Toronto *Evening Telegram* stated: "Assure Bracebridge Nurse Aid in her Cancer 'Cure'. Miss Rene Caisse, With Big Delegation and One-Time Patients, Sees Faulkner." The story reported that Dr. Faulkner had agreed to give Rene Caisse his cooperation in determining the merits of Essiac. "If Miss Caisse has confidence in her cure," the story quoted Faulkner as saying, "she will have a chance to prove it. If it is proved, the government will certainly get behind it."

Dr. Faulkner told the press that he would arrange for Rene to discuss her treatment with Sir Frederick Banting. That was perceived to be a major breakthrough for Rene. Sir Frederick Banting was one of the medical heavyweights of the 1930s, publicly credited as the co-discoverer of insulin, and with his own research facility, The Banting Institute, at the University of Toronto. Faulkner's announcement of Banting's entry into the Essiac controversy made headlines in newspapers all through Canada.

Later in July, 1936, Rene—accompanied by five doctors who supported her work—had her meeting with Dr. Banting. He offered her the facilities of his laboratory and invited her to work there under his supervision performing tests on animals.

"You will not be asked to divulge any secret concerning your treatment," Dr. Banting wrote to Rene on July 23. "All experimental results must be submitted to me for my approval before being announced to anyone, including the newspapers, or published in medical journals."

But there was a catch in Dr. Banting's offer. He wanted Rene to prove the merit of Essiac on the lab animals before she treated any more humans. She would have to give up her work at the clinic for months, or even years, while she injected mice again.

Rene regretfully turned down Sir Frederick Banting. On August 4, 1936, she wrote to Dr. Faulkner explaining her decision: "I have just written to Dr. Banting to tell him that it is impossible for me to accept his kind offer. My relatives and friends do not approve of my going back to animal research, when I have already proven the merit of my Cancer Treatment on human beings.

"Therefore they absolutely refuse to help me financially, and since I have not been able to charge my patients for treatment, I have been at my wits ends to meet the expense of the materials I use. I have never had a hundred dollars I could call my own, therefore it is utterly impossible to do what I haven't the means to do, isn't it? I will just have to go on as I have been doing, and next year I will bring more proof and more names on a petition and we'll make it a political issue.

"I appreciate the fact that you are doing what you think is best for me, and to please you I wish I were in a position to accept this offer, but there is a saying, that you can't get blood out of a stone, and that is my position at the present time."

Dr. Banting wouldn't budge from his position, that Rene could only work on animals in his lab—and nothing else. On the same day she wrote Dr. Faulkner, Dr. Banting wrote the mayor of Bracebridge: "In my opinion it would be impossible for you to adequately test Miss Caisse's cancer treatment in Bracebridge. As I explained to Miss Caisse, I would personally not take any responsibility for work done outside of the laboratory. The whole matter was previously discussed with the Honourable Dr. Faulkner, and we are still prepared to test Miss Caisse's treatment under the arrangements set forth in my letter to her."

Rene wouldn't budge from her position, despite the advice from some of her old allies in the medical world that she might be well advised to consider the offer. Dr. W.C. Arnold wrote to Rene: "I have just read your letter from Banting, and I think it is fair enough. It is the same proposition I made to you many years ago when we put the mice into the Christie Street lab."

While Dr. Arnold agreed that he understood Rene's objections and had some of his own, he wrote that the offer "was, perhaps, as much as you could have expected."

Dr. Banting tried to talk Rene out of her decision, but failed. On August 11, 1936, he wrote her one last time. Implicit in his letter is the belief that her lab tests might well have led to favorable results and his valuable endorsement: "I think you will regret that you have not availed yourself of the offer made by this laboratory. However—if at some future time you again decide to have the treatment investigated, I am sure that Doctor Faulkner and myself would reconsider the matter."

What Dr. Banting really believed about Essiac is nowhere on the record. Rene always maintained that he had told her that what he had seen of Essiac showed more promise than any other cancer treatment he had ever encountered. She said until the end of her life that Dr. Banting had been particularly impressed by one of her cases in which the patient had cancer and diabetes. Since no one knew how Essiac would mix with insulin, the patient's doctor—Dr. J.A. McInnis—had taken the patient off of insulin while the Essiac was administered. The diabetes didn't worsen.

According to Rene, Dr. Banting had been familiar with this case since 1926. He had examined the records and X-rays taken during the Essiac treatments and told Rene that Essiac must have somehow stimulated the pancreatic gland into functioning properly. But only Rene's account of these conversations with Dr. Banting is available today.

More than 40 years after her rejection of Dr. Banting's offer, Rene reminisced to reporters from a Canadian magazine: "He was very kind, but he made it clear I'd have to give up my clinic if I went to work with him. I felt it was inhuman for them to ask me to give up treating patients while I showed them whether it would work on mice. I'd already done work on mice.

"There was a big uproar about it because the patients were terrified I would leave them, but many doctors said I should jump at the chance to work with Dr. Banting. I said I'd be willing to, but I'm not going to let people die while I do it. It was an agonizing decision, but I refused his offer."

Two weeks after Rene turned down Dr. Banting's offer, two New York City cancer specialists arrived in Bracebridge to investigate Rene's work. They liked what they saw, and almost immediately Canadian newspapers carried stories saying that Rene might take her treatment across the border.

On August 27, 1936, the Montreal *Monitor* reported that Rene, "who has become nationally known through her research and interest in the cause of cancer cure and prevention will shortly receive a very attractive offer from American physicians with regard to a position in the United States."

On the same day, the Huntsville *Forester*, decrying this threat from the Americans to steal Rene Caisse away from Canada, editorialized: "If the work of Miss Caisse is the cure of cancer, as is claimed for it, not only should it be welcomed greedily by the medical profession, but it should interest most actively the heads of our health departments of government.

"Evidence of the effectiveness of the treatment given by Miss Caisse seems to be conclusive. Several known cases in Muskoka have been cited where cancer was the professional diagnosis, and where apparent cures have been effected. The patients themselves are the best evidence Miss Caisse can present.

"But instead of a serious attempt being made to capitalize on the discovery of Miss Caisse, the official and professional approach to this matter has been discouragingly technical, skeptical and indifferent. Now, there is a possibility that Bracebridge and Canada may lose Miss Caisse to the more discerning and less rigid medical profession of the United States."

There were other offers from the U.S., and after sorting through her options, Rene finally announced to the press in October, 1936 that she was going to a Chicago university to demonstrate her cancer treatment on some of their patients.

On October 19, the headline in the Toronto *Globe* read: "Cancer Remedy Claimed in Bracebridge Goes to U.S.A." The story reported that Rene was going to be working with a former diagnostician from the Mayo Clinic. The arrangements had been made by a University of Toronto anatomy professor, Dr. B.L. Guyatt, who later became an important supporter in Rene's political fights.

Dr. Guyatt was one of those who visited Rene's clinic to do his own investigation. He wrote in his report: "In most cases distorted countenances became normal and pain reduced as treatment proceeded. The relief from pain is a notable feature, as pain in these cases is very difficult to control.

"The number of patients treated in this clinic are many hundreds and the number responding wholly or in part I do not know, but *I do know* that I have witnessed in this clinic a treatment which brings restoration through destroying the tumor tissue, and supplying that something which improves the mental outlook on life."

At the news that Rene was going to the United States, there was a flood of angry mail to Premier Hepburn and the Minister of Health. The Mayor of Bracebridge wrote to Dr. Faulkner in blunt terms: "The people in this part of the Province who have known of this work are up in arms about the way in which Miss Caisse has been treated."

There were angry editorials in newspapers all through Ontario. And Rene was skillful in her dealings with the press. She was always good for a juicy quote, a quick few lines that would inspire the growing public indignation with the way she was being treated by the Canadian government.

One paper quoted her as saying: "I have been begging the Ontario authorities for thirteen years to give me a chance. I wanted to keep this discovery Canadian, but there seems no chance of bringing out anything of benefit here. I am simply forced to go over to the other side to get recognition."

But she promised that she would never abandon Canada and her patients. She would go to the States only every other week, while maintaining her work at home the rest of the time. "I can assure you that there will always be a cancer clinic in Bracebridge," she told the reporter.

For the next several months, Rene somehow managed the stress of working on both sides of the border. Under the supervision of Dr. John Wolfer, the director of the Tumor Clinic of the Northwestern University Medical School, Rene commuted almost weekly between Chicago and Bracebridge. While keeping her clinic open, she was treating 30 terminally ill patients in Chicago. Five Northwestern doctors were working with her on the project.

In later years she told friends and reporters that the workload during that period was a nightmare. She treated her Bracebridge patients on the weekends, stopped in Toronto to treat a few patients there, then went to Chicago and back to Bracebridge to start all over. She was staying up most of the night in Bracebridge cooking and preparing new batches of Essiac.

At one point she had to beg off her duties in Chicago. She'd made herself sick trying to satisfy everyone's needs. On February 26, 1937, she wrote to Dr. Wolfer: "I am really ill. I treated two hundred patients here at my Clinic a week ago, went on to Toronto and treated fourteen more, then on to Walkerville to treat again more.

"When I took ill, my brother-in-law from Ferndale, Michigan came after me in a car and took me to my sister who had her family doctor see me. He said it was my heart and over-nervous strain and that I need two or three months absolute rest.

"But tomorrow I must start on my patients here again. I wanted to please you, but it was unfair of you to have me spend about a hundred dollars besides risking my health to go there and treat six patients, for you, as I did last time I was there. Tell me candidly if you have lost interest."

He hadn't. He wrote Rene back on March 13, 1937, saying he was slow to respond because he'd been out of the country, and he was still "in hopes that we might be able to carry along our work at the Clinic for a sufficient time to provide us with some evidence to enable us to make up our minds relative to your treatment."

Before long, Rene was feeling well enough to return to Chicago and carry on as before. On March 25, she wrote Dr. Wolfer to say she would be back on April 4. He wrote her back immediately saying he was glad to hear the news and would make the arrangements.

Rene's return was brief. She soon got sick again and decided she'd better stay in Bracebridge. But one of the doctors in Chicago, Dr. Clifford Barbouka, had seen enough to be a believer. He offered her facilities at Chicago's Passavant Hospital if she wanted to move there. But she chose to stay at home in Bracebridge.

When the news that she was too ill to travel reached her patients in Chicago, at least one of them was alarmed enough to write directly to Rene. On May 14, 1937, May Miller of Chicago wrote to say she hoped Rene was recovering from her latest illness and to say she hoped she'd be seeing Rene again.

"The first time I came to the Northwestern University Tumor Clinic to receive your arm injections," Ms. Miller wrote, "I had been for several weeks previous, suffering such acute agony in my shoulder, back of my neck, and up in the back of my head, that my doctor had given me a narcotic to enable me to rest some at night.

"So when, shortly before the fifth injection, I realized that the terrible head pain at the back had subsided and that though I still had pain, it was in such a lesser degree (I have to take anidon (sic) pain tablets for it) and I was starting to get some sleep at night, I was mighty thankful to God because of your coming to this Clinic here.

"Miss Case (sic), since I was starting to feel much better of my pain, wouldn't I have felt practically none pain by now, if it had not been that you were stricken with your two severe illnesses and so could not give us the benefit of your injections?

"About three weeks ago my neck swelling suddenly began to pain considerably. It makes me hope we'll be seeing you soon again, for I am sure I was being helped."

By now, the Canadian press was making a political issue out of Rene Caisse and Essiac. At the beginning of 1937, with Rene's work on both sides of the border getting attention, the Toronto *Evening Telegram* set the tone for the coming debate with an editorial comparing the government's treatment of Rene with the hostility Louis Pasteur had faced in an earlier century. "It is to be questioned whether to-day the medical profession has brought a sufficiently open mind to its fight against cancer."

Saying that Rene was "reported to have attained astonishing results," the *Telegram* knocked the medical authorities for their attitude of "Put your formula on the table and we will tell you whether we will help you."

Dr. Banting, the paper said, "did not place insulin on the table until he was satisfied with the results of his research....If it is a fact that a clinic has been provided in Chicago and refused in Ontario, it is necessary that there should be an explanation of the reason for the refusal here. Results are more important than medical etiquette."

Angry letters from citizens began to pour into the offices of the Minister of Health and the Prime Minister of Ontario, Mitchell Hepburn. Typical of the mail Hepburn was receiving was the letter he received from a nurse in Peterboro, Ontario, who was caring for one of Rene's patients and had seen the benefits of Essiac.

The patient, Mrs. Oliver, had been operated on in November, 1936. The surgeon had found a cancerous growth on her colon, which he couldn't remove. "Nothing could be done for her, just a matter of time, possibly six months," the nurse wrote. "Meaning another life gone. When she came home from the hospital hardly able to walk across the floor and suffering from such severe pain that she could neither sleep nor rest was when I came to care for her."

Mrs. Oliver's husband had heard of Nurse Caisse and as the only chance, they took Mrs. Oliver to Bracebridge. "She has now had 4 treatments & improving all the time. Everyone marvels at the change in her. Now Hon. Premier Hepburn, does it seem fair to you to make it so that Miss Caisse may no longer give treatments when hundreds of outcast patients from the foremost hospitals and noted doctors are at the present depending on her treatments for life? Does it seem fair to you that the formula should be taken from Miss Caisse to experiment on guinea pigs when it has been tried and proven successful on hundreds of human beings? Who is foremost in this Prov. of Ont., human beings or guinea pigs? When Drs. admit that they are unable to cure or do anything for patients why take from someone that which is proving successful?"

Passions were running high. The government was being forced into a position where it had to do something. They had to put Rene out of business, arrest her, get her formula, or finally authorize her to practice medicine.

On March 8, 1937, the Toronto *Evening Telegram* reported: "Matters soon will reach a final stage in the efforts of Miss Rene Caisse, Bracebridge nurse, to obtain Canadian medical recognition for her cancer treatment methods." The story said that next week a large deputation from various locations in Ontario would be calling on Premier Hepburn and Dr. Faulkner and other cabinet members. They would urge that she be given the right to practice medicine, and they would be carrying a new petition—this one with 14,000 signatures.

The deputation, the paper reported, would include several doctors, notably Dr. B.L. Guyatt of the University of Toronto, Dr. W.C. Arnold, Dr. Herbert Minthorn—the associate coroner of two Ontario districts—and Dr. J.A. McInnis.

A few nights before the group left for Toronto, the mayor of Bracebridge organized a town meeting to rally support. The high school gymnasium was packed. The mayor told the crowd that the vast sums of money spent on cancer research had produced no recognized cures. He said he didn't know if Rene Caisse had a cure, but he did know that people who were suffering from cancer before they went to Rene were well today.

Dr. Edward Ellis told the crowd that he had seen interesting results from Rene's treatments, but that "science creeps slowly. We can only think so much and say little as doctors, although as private citizens we are right behind a beneficial treatment."

Dr. Minthorn stood up and said that he had seen Rene's work three times four weeks apart. He was skeptical at first. "But Miss Caisse is doing a good work and has ample proof."

Rene's long-time supporter, Dr. J.A. McInnis, told of his acquaintance with Rene, dating back to when only a few people knew what she was doing. "Personally," he told the crowd, "I am absolutely convinced that Miss Caisse's methods will arrest pain, reduce cancer growth and prolong life, and I say that very guardedly."

Some of Rene's patients told their own stories. Jack Vanclieaf walked to the platform and said: "Here I am alive today, while I would have been dead years ago had it not been for Miss Caisse. Two good doctors told me I had only two months to live. I went to Miss Caisse and within three days the intense pain was relieved and with more treatments I kept on getting better. Hon. Dr. Faulkner told me I hadn't cancer, but all I've to say is, what is the difference between being eaten by a wolf or eaten by a bear? The doctor said he couldn't cure me and that I would die. Miss Caisse cured me in six treatments."

The deputation that went to the government offices in Toronto consisted of local officials, 40 doctors and 18 of Rene's patients. They were carrying a petition that now had 17,000 signatures. Things were moving fast. There were more front page headlines throughout Ontario when the Minister of Health, Dr. Faulkner, and Dr. R. T. Noble of the College of Physicians and Surgeons met with the group. Later in the day Sir Frederick Banting met with some of them.

After the meetings, Dr. Faulkner told the press: "We are considering introducing legislation that will give all the people who have the idea they have a cure for cancer an opportunity to submit their cures to test and they will receive such encouragement that will put beyond doubt the nature of the treatment."

That was the first time a public official had mentioned legislation to deal with the situation. Public pressure was great enough that the battle was now working its way toward the Canadian parliament.

In July, 1937, with an election coming up in a few months and the letters pouring in from Rene's patients and supporters, Premier Mitchell Hepburn agreed to meet her in his Queens Park office. Rene told the press the Premier had been encouraging. Talking about Rene and her supporters, Premier Hepburn told the press: "These people are sincere, clear-thinking people, and it seems to me that something must be done to make this treatment available to all people suffering from cancer.

"The onus is now on the medical profession. They must now either prove or disprove Miss Caisse's claims, and I do not believe they can disprove them. I am in sympathy with Miss Caisse's work, and will do all in my power to help her."

He stated publicly that if he had to, he would see that a bill licensing her to practice would be passed in the legislature.

Politically, that put Hepburn way out in front of cautious politicians and skeptical doctors. No such bill allowing one private citizen without the proper medical credentials to practice medicine had ever been passed in the history of Canada. But Hepburn had seen enough mail and heard from enough of Rene's patients to know that the public was solidly behind her. He knew where the votes were.

At the same time, a group of American businessmen from Buffalo, New York, had become familiar with Essiac and they drew up a contract and presented it to Rene. For the right to represent Essiac in the U.S., they promised to pay her at least $100,000 in the first year, $50,000 in all succeeding years, plus 50% "of all sums received" from the use of Essiac. In a separate letter to her a few weeks later, their lawyer, Ralph Saft, sweetened the offer by promising a $1 million "donation" to her work.

Rene had meetings with them and extensive correspondence. But she gradually became convinced that they were only out to make a fast buck. She was afraid they would exploit the rich and make Essiac prohibitively expensive for the poor. She turned them down and stuck their contract in her files, alongside the one she'd been offered by the businessman from Toronto.

By mid-1937, hundreds of people a week desperate for Rene's help were flocking to her clinic. She was treating as many of them as possible, still staying up half the night in her kitchen brewing the Essiac, but she was now beginning to face a new problem. An increasing number of patients were arriving without a signed letter from a physician stating a diagnosis of cancer. Some doctors—fearful of offending Canada's powerful College of Physicians and Surgeons—were refusing to put into writing this release Rene was required to have before treating anyone.

This new obstacle caused scenes and dramatically added to Rene's stress, as she dealt with how to prod the doctors into action, how to stall the frantic patients, even how to treat people without the necessary documentation and still avoid jail.

But the hostility of much of the medical establishment didn't prevent the most solid citizens from seeking out Rene. The president of the Toronto *Globe and Mail* newspaper sent one of his own staffers to be treated by Rene.

A lawyer in Des Moines, Iowa, wrote to Rene saying that his college roommate's wife had been cured of breast cancer by Essiac and the lawyer now wanted to make arrangements for Rene to treat another friend of his, an Iowa Supreme Court Justice.

A woman physician from Los Angeles, Dr. Emma Carson, who had heard accounts of Rene's successes, traveled from southern California to Bracebridge in the summer of 1937 to see for herself.

She later told reporters that she had been skeptical, even though her friends who had told her about Rene were reliable people. Intending only to stay in Bracebridge for a couple of days to satisfy herself that there was nothing to the story, she ended up staying almost a month and becoming a good friend of Rene's.

In Dr. Carson's first interview, with the Huntsville *Forester* a week after her arrival, she could barely contain her enthusiasm. "I am simply amazed at what I have found in my already brief investigation," she said. "The farther I investigate, the stronger becomes my conviction that Miss Caisse has made a cancer treatment discovery of world-wide importance."

Dr. Carson said that she had found "some amazing cases." She called upon the government to recognize Rene Caisse's work. "If in view of what I have seen with my own eyes, the Ontario Medical Council remains indifferent, it will be a crime against civilization." She said that when she finished her investigation, she would go directly to Prime Minister Hepburn's office and give him her report.

Dr. Carson never changed her mind about Rene Caisse and Essiac. She kept up her correspondence with Rene for years after she returned to Los Angeles, and when she had concluded her investigation she wrote a five-page report and released it to the press. Several newspapers quoted all or much of what she had to say.

"The vast majority of Miss Caisse's patients," Dr. Carson wrote, "were brought to her after surgery, radium, X-rays, emplastrums, etc., had failed to be helpful and the patients were pronounced incurable or hopeless cases. The progress obtainable and the actual results from Essiac treatments, and the rapidity of repair were absolutely marvelous, and must be seen to be believed." As she reviewed case histories and interviewed patients, she wrote, "I realized that skepticism had deserted me."

In November, Hepburn's Liberal Party won the elections, and Rene received a friendly note from Hepburn's secretary saying that if Rene would like another meeting with the Prime Minister, please just advise them by telephone.

In less than three years, Rene Caisse had gone from being an obscure nurse in the northwoods treating those people in the area who'd heard of her by word of mouth to a national figure in Canada, with an open door in the office of the Prime Minister of Ontario. She was the center of a major political controversy. Her thousands of backers were passionate about her cause, especially those who had been her patients.

From the beginning, the people who had been treated with Essiac were the ones who spread the word, wrote the press, wrote the politicians, sent Rene more patients, and pushed the government to legalize her practice.

All through Rene's files are testimonials from her patients, dating from the 1920s to the 1970s. They are anecdotal and written by laymen with no medical training. But there are so many, from every level of society in the U.S. and Canada, and the people who wrote them were so deeply affected and so passionate in their belief, that after reading through all of them, they become impossible to ignore.

Many of these statements are so categorical that if they are even close to portraying accurately what happened, they alone should be enough to prompt serious scientific curiosity about this herbal blend called Essiac.

As 1937 ended, Rene's supporters were rallying for the big push in 1938. Politically, 1938 would tell the tale. The cause had reached parliament, and the legislators were going to have to face the issue of Essiac, one way or the other. In the course of organizing their campaign, several of Rene's former patients took the step of swearing their stories under oath.

One of those testimonials is an affidavit sworn on December 7, 1937, by a man named Henry J. Hneeshaw. To confirm part of what he said, Mr. Hneeshaw submitted a letter from the Mayo Clinic, signed by George B. Eusterman. "At the time you were here we found you to have an inoperable gastric carcinoma," the letter said. "Roentgenoscopic examination showed extensive involvement, including the upper third. Gastric analysis disclosed an anacidity and other evidence of involvement of the upper third of the stomach. We would not recommend surgical exploration."

Mr. Hneeshaw attached to the letter what he swore as true. Here's what he said: For a year, he suffered stomach discomfort and severe loss of appetite. On May 25, 1937, he went to his doctor, who examined him and suspected cancer. After examination by four other doctors in a cancer clinic, Mr. Hneeshaw was told that he had cancer of the stomach. On June 4, he went into surgery. "But after opening me they decided not to operate as the growth was right into the diaphragm and operation would be fatal. They gave me three months to live."

He went home and was losing weight rapidly. At the end of July, he went to the Mayo Clinic after hearing that they could do wonderful things for cancer patients. After five days, they told him nothing could be done.

Mr. Hneeshaw had heard of Miss Caisse. "As a final effort to live I thought it could do no harm to see her. I cannot express my gratitude and appreciation at what she has done. I had my first treatment from her on August ninth, and from that first treatment I felt a different man. I weighed then 129 pounds, now weigh 150 pounds and am better in every way. The discomfort is almost gone and I can eat and enjoy my food. I feel stronger all the time and am looking forward to farming out West just as good as ever."

Every day, statements like that were arriving in the offices of legislators and the Minister of Health and the Ontario Prime Minister. They were running in the letters to the editor columns of newspapers. The politicians knew that this was not going to be an easy matter to deal with.

Rene Caisse was hopeful that 1938 would be the year that Essiac won the official acceptance and legal authorization that she— and her supporters—passionately believed it deserved. But whatever was going to happen, she was going to make one hell of a fight of it.

CHAPTER
THREE

Probably not even Rene could have imagined the fight that she would live through in 1938. She was in the newspapers regularly all year. In small ways and large, tens of thousands of people involved themselves in her cause. At one point, Ontario Prime Minister Mitchell Hepburn received yet another petition on Rene's behalf—this one with 55,000 signatures.

Hundreds of people a week were showing up at her clinic, most of them desperately ill. Her former patients were still spreading the word about their treatments. To understand the phenomenon that Rene had become in Canada, it's necessary to understand what her patients were going around telling people.

A woman named E.A. Tarzwell from Milton, Ontario read about Rene in a newspaper that published a letter from one of Rene's patients, James Summerwill, a notary public in Sprucedale, Ontario. Mrs. Tarzwell wrote directly to Mr. Summerwill to find out more. These were strangers corresponding about matters of life and death, and there was no reluctance, no equivocation, in what Mr. Summerwill wrote back to Mrs. Tarzwell, based on his own experience.

"As we have passed through the ordeal which you are now experiencing," he wrote to her, "our sincere sympathy is yours. But let me assure you that you have no cause to worry over more than the actual suffering of your husband, providing that the trouble is not too much advanced, if he is taking Miss Caisse's treatment and follows her instructions completely."

He told of his case. He was suffering from "the most malignant type of cancer known." Dr. Faulkner, Premier Hepburn's Minister of Health in the previous cabinet, had personally told him that Dr. Faulkner had never heard of anyone being cured of Mr. Summerwill's type of cancer. Mr. Summerwill's doctors told him that surgery was the only hope. He refused the surgery and got his doctor to write the necessary consent letter to allow Rene to treat him.

"I took 28 treatments in all, weekly, 1 treatment until the last 2 which was 1 treatment semi-weekly. My cancer was in the left groin. From the 5th treatment I could notice a slight improvement at the end of each week, which gave me a little encouragement, and I persevered and gained very slowly but surely. I took my last treatment 24th June, 1936, and have been feeling fine ever since and able to look after my work from that time. But of course I had to take things easy for quite a while in order not to put too much strain on the parts that had been afflicted."

Mr. Summerwill concluded his letter: "At this time there is not the least sign of a return of the trouble. I take the time and trouble to answer a very large number of letters along the same line as yours for the reason that I would like everyone suffering that terrible affliction to receive at least relief and a 90% chance of a cure."

He attached to his letter a carbon copy of his doctor's diagnosis:"Lymphosarcoma."

Try to imagine, fifty years later, the kind of public sensation that was caused by all sorts of testimonials like that published in newspapers and with similar letters pouring into the offices of legislators and Premier Hepburn. The son of Ontario's Senator Marshall was telling all his friends that this nurse in Bracebridge was curing cancer. One legislator wrote to Rene on January 22, 1938, to offer any legislative help he could give—and to ask for three bottles of Essiac.

A woman named Eva Stephens wrote Premier Hepburn a long and articulate letter explaining how Rene Caisse had cured her when the doctors had failed. In passing, she mentioned: "I was in Miss Caisse's clinic the other day when a lady was discharged fully cured from cancer of the breast and even our medical doctors can find no trace of cancer. I wish you could have talked to that lady."

Rene herself wasn't mincing any words in her correspondence with the politically powerful. On February 14, 1938, she gave Premier Hepburn a piece of her mind. After bluntly pointing out that her endorsement had helped his campaign the previous fall, she took him to task for denying to the Toronto *Daily Star* that he had promised to put a bill through the legislature granting her a special license to practice.

"When I told you that the Medical Assocation was very powerful," she wrote, "your answer to me was, 'they are not as strong as our legislature.' Now, if you have found out that the Medical Profession is more powerful than you thought it was, and have found that your hands are tied and that you cannot keep your promise to me, would it not have been more manly or more kindly to have admitted that you were unable to keep your promise, than to publicly deny having made it, making me out untruthful?"

Hepburn relented. The Toronto newspapers later reported that he had arranged for Rene's special bill to be introduced in the legislature a week later. Accompanied by a list of names of more than 200 former patients who swore they had benefited from Essiac, the bill, if passed, would grant that: "Rene Caisse be authorized to practice medicine in the Province of Ontario in the treatment of cancer in all its forms and of human ailments and conditions resulting therefrom."

In response, the organized medical opposition lowered the boom. After the 1937 election, Dr. Faulkner had left his post as Minister of Health and been replaced by Harold Kirby. At the beginning of March, the "Kirby Bill" was introduced in the legislature.

The Kirby Bill was advertised to the public as a way of getting to the truth about Rene's treatment, and a handful of other controversial cancer treatments then in use in Canada.

To protect the public and discover if any of these treatments had merit, the Kirby Bill would authorize the establishment of a Royal Cancer Commission to investigate all possible cancer cures.

Rene, of course, would be allowed to offer evidence to the Royal Cancer Commission, to be composed of respected members of the Canadian College of Physicians and Surgeons. If her evidence were persuasive, the Cancer Commission would legalize Essiac.

But there was a catch. The formulas for all treatments investigated would have to be turned over to the Cancer Commission. Anyone refusing to divulge their formula could be fined $100 to $500 the first time they were caught treating a patient; and $500 to $2,500 the second time, and for each subsequent offense. Failure to pay the fine could result in 30 days to six months in jail. Harsh measures, indeed.

According to the Kirby Bill, the members of the Cancer Commission would be required to maintain the confidentiality of the formula for any cancer treatment. But there were no penalties attached to their failure to do so.

Rene told friends that if the Kirby Bill passed and she turned over the formula, every secretary and doctor who got hold of it could—and probably would—do whatever they pleased with it, with no fear of punishment. She was outraged at this obvious insult to her.

Dismissing any possibility the Cancer Commission would keep her formula secret, Rene told the press: "The people of Ontario will be paying a group of men to develop something that was developed and discovered 15 years ago. I have developed and proven a cure right here in Bracebridge, and I am running a clinic where hundreds of cancer sufferers are being treated and helped. Why then should I be asked to give my formula over to a group of doctors who never did anything to earn it?"

The press reported that 28,000 signatures were now on a petition that would soon be submitted to parliament in support of Rene's bill. "I would certainly welcome any committee sent here by the government," Rene told reporters. But if the Kirby Bill passed, she threatened, she would have no choice but to leave the country. "If the Ontario legislature can pass a law to put me in jail for six months for helping suffering people, I will close my clinic and go to the United States. I shall not buck such opposition." On March 10, 1938, Rene's threat made headlines in the Toronto newspapers. Meanwhile Rene's backers were lobbying with fervor. But these were not, for the most part, powerful and well-connected people. One of their main weapons had to be the letters they wrote to the people who were.

Within days of the introduction of the Kirby Bill, Rene's backers organized a massive campaign of letters to legislators and potential witnesses for Essiac. On March 11, Mrs. D.A. Heimbecker of Bracebridge wrote that she couldn't make it to Toronto as a delegate but wanted to add her letter to the campaign.

"I had two operations about seven years ago for cancer," she wrote to one of the women who was organizing the lobbying effort. "After a few years the trouble came back. My Dr. couldn't help me, so I just lived thinking I would have to die in a few years. So last summer I heard of Miss Rene Caisse of Bracebridge. I came here last October 12, 1937, and after I had my third treatment I knew that she could help me. I am still taking treatments but I know that I am cured. But a few more treatments wouldn't hurt. I certainly feel like a new person thanks to Miss Rene Caisse for my health."

On March 14, Mrs. John Thornbury wrote her simple statement to the same organizer: An X-ray had indicated that she needed an operation, but she was too weak. "I was so weak I was not able to walk alone. My husband had to carry me for months and I could not eat anything and could not even keep a drink down. I started to go up to Miss Caisse for treatments in July and now I am feeling fine and have a good appetite and can do a good lot of my own work and I know I have sure been benefited by Miss Caisse's treatments. And I think I can say I am almost cured. Yours truly."

On March 15, a woman named Ann Mitchell from Milford Bay, Ontario wrote her "To whom it may concern" contribution. In a long and vivid letter, she told a horrifying story of one cancer after another being removed by surgery and treated with radium. But they kept coming back. Finally when the cancer returned again, she refused radium. "I was so burned and sick from this I decided to give Miss Caisse a trial and I am only sorry I didn't go sooner as I would have saved a good bit of suffering and expense."

Rene treated Ann Mitchell from March to July, 1937. She gained 20 pounds and returned to normal health. Describing her experiences at Rene's clinic, she wrote: "From week to week I've seen great changes in many poor sick people. If anything I could say or do to help Miss Caisse I'd certainly be glad to do it."

Rene's supporters gathered piles of letters like this, from people all over Canada, many of them total strangers to each other who had no way of knowing what others were writing, who had nothing to gain by their statements, and who all told similar stories. Not even the most skeptical—or hostile—legislator could dismiss Rene out of hand with this kind of record compiled.

In the third week of March, the Private Bills committee of the Ontario legislature considered the bill that would authorize Rene Caisse to treat cancer patients with Essiac. The petition with 55,000 signatures was presented to them. Fifty of Rene's patients watched from the visitor's gallery.

The debate was fierce. J. Frank Kelly, the MP from the Bracebridge area and an ardent backer of Rene's, argued that she had been "hounded around the country for years like a criminal. I'm not claiming that Miss Caisse has a cancer cure. But I know people who were sick and are well today, and I know that their illness was diagnosed as cancer by the medical profession. Even if she hasn't a cure for cancer but can prolong life, she should get some consideration. Even Sir Frederick Banting does not pretend to be able to cure diabetes with insulin, but he can prolong life and relieve suffering."

"But isn't she carrying on now?" a committee member named L.M. Frost asked.

"Yes, she's carrying on but without fee and without recognition. I don't know whether the committee wants to go so far as to make her a doctor but she should get some sort of recognition. Give her a chance to carry on helping people."

Rene's lawyer, John Carrick, claimed that "patients and their relatives are reporting that doctors are refusing to give her diagnoses of cancer, and that a cabal has been organized by the medical profession against her."

Some MP's shouted "Untrue" and "Shame." At that, one of Rene's patients stood up and yelled out: "My mother was a cancer patient, yet three doctors refused to give her a written diagnosis for Miss Caisse, though they gave it to my mother verbally."

The patients in the gallery cheered and applauded, prompting Speaker David Croll to threaten to have them removed. John Carrick then read the case of James Summerwill, the notary public who claimed to have been cured of lymphosarcoma, into the record and said, "I have many patients here willing to speak to the committee if they are wanted."

Speaker Croll declined that opportunity. "The government is setting up a board to deal with these reported cures," he said, referring to the Cancer Commission to be established if the Kirby Bill passed.

But another MP, William Duckworth from Toronto, said that Rene's patients should be heard. Pointing to the visitor's gallery, he said: "We have to take their word." The gallery erupted in cheers.

Dr. M.T. Armstrong, the MP from Parry Sound, spoke in support of the bill. "I don't know whether it's a cure or not," he said, "but I certainly have seen people who have been helped by her. I've talked to practically every medical doctor in the legislature, and there isn't one who's against her."

Another MP from Toronto, W.A. Summerville, said that he'd heard from all sorts of people who claimed to have been helped by Rene Caisse. "We want to help suffering humanity. What Miss Caisse wants is protection. This committee should do something to protect her."

Then William Duckworth added: "She should be helped. The Minister (of Health) says that the Health Department has not interfered with Miss Caisse. Well, I say that heads of the department change. They may be gone in two or three years."

There was an argument about whether doctors were for Rene Caisse or against her, and whether this bill was a premature stamp of approval or merely a way to allow her to continue without interference until science could determine the truth about Essiac.

A man named T.F. Stevenson, whose wife had been treated by Rene, was allowed to speak. He said that his wife had not been cured but her pain had been diminished. He made an impassioned plea for the bill. "Why hold this woman up? You won't do any harm by passing this bill and it's inhuman to stop it. Let her go for the sake of humanity, even if she can only give relief from pain. Then at least cancer sufferers can die in peace without the aid of opiates, which is all the medical profession can give them."

Then Rene spoke. She charged that doctors were having the clamps put on them so that they would not give diagnoses to people who wanted to be treated by Rene. "The fact that I can get any results at all should be accepted as a great thing," she said. "When I had success, I thought the doctors would welcome me with open arms. I didn't anticipate antagonism from the profession. I expected cooperation and I have every respect for the profession."

She declared that she would give her formula to the world without any thought of gain "if I knew that it would be given to humanity in the same way. I have never asked a patient for one cent. I have been glad to have donations of $1 or $2 but I have never asked a patient if they had money. I treated them whether they had it or not."

She said that she would happily submit her formula to any investigating commission, on one condition: That the medical profession would admit that Essiac had merit, based on the results she had already obtained. Then she welcomed any sort of investigation of her work. "My clinic is wide open to any investigation at all times."

According to newspaper accounts, when the time for a vote came, there was confusion and many voices speaking at once and a flood of motions to the chairman. Then the chairman recognized a motion that "the bill be not reported," and a show of hands indicated a narrow margin in favor of rejecting the bill. The newspapers reported that Rene's bill had been defeated by three votes.

Rene's hometown paper, the Bracebridge *Gazette*, gave this account on March 31, 1938: "Miss Rene Caisse got kind of turned down by a Parliamentary Committee last week. They put it off on the grounds that a bill covering all such cases is to be introduced, but they did promise that she would not be molested while working as she has been.

"It is difficult to understand the tyrannical treatment Miss Caisse has received. She has been treating people with cancerous growths for fifteen years. In recent years the town of Bracebridge gave her the use of The British Lion, a good brick hotel building.

"There she has treated hundreds of cancer sufferers. Many of these came to her in such condition that there was no possible hope of restoration, but even they had their last days practically free from pain.

"Others who were not so bad, but some of them very bad, have gone away to all appearances cured. At the meeting of a Parliamentary Committee many of these cured persons were present. So enthusiastic was their demonstration in favor of Miss Caisse that officers threatened to clear the room.

"On the other hand among the hundreds who have been treated by Miss Caisse there has never been noted an instance where her treatment has harmed a patient. It is common knowledge that cancers have been cured, at least temporarily, by radium and the knife but those have failed in many times the proportion in which they have succeeded.

"When therefore it is an undisputed fact that Miss Caisse's treatment has never done harm and has so often done good, even to the saving of life, it is difficult to realize the mentality of those who would put obstacles in her way.

"Miss Caisse is not strong and has worked very hard under a very great strain. She will be away from her clinic for a month for absolute rest, leaving no address."

Within days the legislature passed the Kirby Bill into law, and thus began one of the strangest—even bizarre—phases of Rene's battles with the Canadian government. Reduced to its simplest terms, Rene would announce to the press that, because of the Kirby Bill, she was closing her clinic. The press and the public would flock to Kirby's door. Kirby would say no, the law wasn't being enforced, she should open her clinic. Rene would open the clinic. Then someone would frighten her that Kirby was coming after her. She'd close the clinic. The press and the public would...And so it went for the better part of the next two years.

Rene fired first at the end of March. After a few weeks of rest and under heavy pressure from patients and supporters, she announced—to front page headlines—that she would reopen on April 30. Four weeks later, days before the Kirby Bill went into effect, she announced she was closing again.

The Bracebridge *Gazette* reported that her announcement caused "widespread regret in Muskoka and elsewhere....The general opinion in Muskoka is that this statute is arbitrary and unfair. The general feeling here is that the sole test of her treatment should be 'Does it cure?' and that if it cures it should be nobody's business 'how' or 'why' it cures....The probable result of the new legislation will be that Miss Caisse's treatment will be given in the United States and not in Ontario. How do Muskoka cancer sufferers like this prospect?"

Harold Kirby felt enough heat from those people that he called in the press. "KIRBY DENIES NURSE FORCED TO SHUT CLINIC," said the front page headline in the Toronto *Globe and Mail*. "Replies to Protest."

Then he gave reporters a copy of the letter he had written to Rene's lawyer. The Cancer Commission, he said in the letter, will have the authority, after finishing its investigation, to compel Rene to turn over her formula. In the meantime: "It should be made clear to everyone that nothing in this Act prevents Miss Caisse from carrying on with her clinic as she has been doing in the past." Rene was in the same position now, he said, that she was before the passing of the bill.

Nonsense, snapped Rene. Dr. Noble of the College of Physicians and Surgeons, she told reporters, had informed her that they were going to demand her formula if she kept the clinic open. "I regret with all my heart closing my cancer clinic here at Bracebridge. I have battled with the medical profession but when it comes to fighting the law of the Province it is too much for me."

The Huntsville *Forester* later described the scene when the patients at Rene's clinic were notified of the closing: "Tears began to flow down the cheeks of dozens of cancer victims, who had been receiving benefit from their treatment with Miss Caisse, and whose last hope apparently vanished with the announcement of the closing of the clinic. One patient is reported to have fainted, while others, in complete dejection, had to be assisted to their motor cars. Miss Caisse herself was so overcome that she had to leave the scene."

The story quoted three of Rene's patients saying they had been given up for dead by their doctors before Rene's Caisse's treatments had saved their lives. One man told the paper that his wife had been making encouraging progress until the clinic closed. Then she gave up hope and said he "might as well take her home to die."

The story reported that a contingent of these patients and their friends and families went straight to the offices of the area's mayors, who in turn fired off angry telegrams to Premier Hepburn.

The angry letters poured into Kirby's and Hepburn's offices. Typical of what Kirby heard from the public was this, dated May 30,1938, from Mr. J.M. Andercheck of Timmons, Ontario: "It has been a very severe blow to me as well as to many of the sufferers to hear that Miss Caisse was forced to close her clinic. I think it is a great injustice to the hundreds of sufferers from the dreadful disease whom Miss Caisse has so greatly benefited.

"My wife was one of her patients for the last 3 months and has gained in health and confidence and was looking forward to regaining her health again.

"She is only 34 years of age and a mother of a 3-year-old child. It seems such a pity to take away the opportunity from a person her age to regain her health and happiness to which every person is entitled to. And leave nothing but despair."

Those who were devastated by the closing of the clinic poured out their feelings in letters to Rene. In one that conveys beautifully the feelings of those who had been treated with Essiac, William Giles wrote: "Your tragic message received. As I sit here, I am picturing the crowds of sad, pathetic faces whose only hope in life was through Miss Caisse.

"What a Godsend you were to us all. Whatever will we do without you girls. Just sit back to brood and die in despair. You were helping us so much & now there seems to be no other way out of our difficulties. However, where jealous, covetous doctors have made this Rich Blessing impossible for Canadians, we trust & hope that your wonderful services will continue on to help, encourage & cure our sister nation, the Americans. We often wonder at it all but I doubt if we shall ever quite understand....You made things so nice & easy for us. We can never forget you. Goodbye with love and every good wish."

Rene's supporters were quickly organizing their counterattack. On May 30, one of them sent out a mass mailing to all of Rene's patients: "We may find it necessary to take a delegation to Queen's Park, in which case we would have to have as large a crowd as possible. We are depending on you to join us."

That same day Premier Hepburn sent a telegram to the mayor of Huntsville, Ontario: "This government has taken no action whatsoever to interfere in any way with operation of Miss Caisse's clinic....Would suggest that representations be made to her urging her to continue treatment of those who have confidence in her formula."

Three days later, on June 2, Hepburn wrote directly to Rene. In a two-page letter he gently encouraged her to keep the clinic open and urged her to turn over the formula, if the Cancer Commission requested it. "You have read the statement which was issued to the press," the Premier wrote. "It should be clear to you that no action has been taken by the Government to close your clinic."

The next day's headlines said that Rene was "reassured" by Premier Hepburn's statements and that the clinic would reopen.

But Rene denied the accuracy of those reports. She said that the clinic would remain closed. On June 3, 1938, the Toronto *Evening Telegram* reported that "she could not possibly see her way clear to continue treating her many patients while the law of the province places her in such a position that she cannot be free to carry on her work."

There was a flood of telegrams to Hepburn and Kirby. More petitions were circulated and signed. Angry Ontario newspapers editorialized on Rene's behalf. Typical of the editorials was this in the Orangeville *Banner*: "Miss Caisse is liable to a penalty if she refuses to disclose her formula. On the other hand members of the Commission and their clerks are protected by the Act, even if they disclose the formula inadvertently or deliberately. It is a piece of unfair, one-sided legislation, quite unworthy of a deliberative body representing the people of Ontario.

"It is difficult to retain one's respect for a Legislature that placed such an unfair and one-sided Act on the statute books of this province. Under the circumstances it is not surprising that Miss Caisse has decided to close her clinic and seek in the United States the freedom that is denied her in her own province."

On June 16, the Toronto *Evening Telegram* reported that Hepburn and Kirby had been "besieged with letters from patients who have beeen deprived of their treatments."

That same day there was another announcement that the clinic would reopen. Then on June 20, the Toronto newspapers reported that Kirby had repudiated his negotiations with Rene's lawyers and the clinic would remain closed.

There was another public outcry. On June 23, the Toronto *Evening Telegram* reported the story of "a Toronto woman with fear in her eyes" who "begs" the *Telegram*: "Please do what you can to get the clinic re-opened. It means my life."

According to the *Evening Telegram*, the woman had a medical diagnosis of inoperable cancer of the stomach. She told the paper that two months earlier, out of desperation, she had gone to the Caisse clinic. "Three treatments, one a week, improved me tremendously," the paper quoted her as saying. "I felt like a different person, and my doctor expressed amazement and said he wouldn't have believed it possible."

She told the paper that she was "terribly, terribly anxious to continue these treatments." But when she phoned Bracebridge for an appointment, "Miss Caisse said she was afraid to re-open. I cannot understand for the life of me—and it means my life— why the government cannot let doctors diagnose cancer cases, have Miss Caisse treat them, and judge her discovery by cures. That should be proof enough. While they're making a political football out of this what is going to happen to people like me? Our time is—limited."

The *Evening Telegram* described this unnamed woman as the "wife of a man in a responsible business position, of comfortable means."

When she finished telling her own story, she described for the paper her encounters with some of Rene's other patients: "A little old lady had a bunch of violets in her hand. She said she had picked them herself for Miss Caisse—she who had cancer of the stomach and could not walk when she first went to her for treatments. There was another woman of 28, from Capreol, mother of three small children. She had been twice operated on for cancer of the throat and her vocal chords had been cut, so that she could speak only in a whisper. She whispered to me: 'I've gained 13 pounds since coming here, and the pain has gone from my throat.' I wonder what that poor thing is doing with her treatments cut off."

The paper said that this woman did not blame Rene Caisse for closing her clinic. "She should get credit for it, and should be allowed herself to prove its value," the woman was quoted as saying. "She treats poor and rich alike without question. Some are so poor that they can pay nothing. I saw a countryman with a dozen eggs in payment for a treatment. Everybody gives her what they can afford."

The woman's grown son was quoted speaking bitterly of the Kirby Bill: "Kirby says if they disprove her formula in the medical laboratory, they still can't prevent her operating a clinic," the son said. "What it amounts to, then, is that somebody wants the formula. It's not for the protection of the public, because, according to his own statement, she can run a clinic anyway. If you had seen my mother before the treatments Miss Caisse gave her, you would know there was something in her discovery. Somebody's trying to get it—and get the credit for it."

The story ended by noting: "At Queen's Park, warm denial is reiterated that Miss Caisse has any reason 'to be afraid' to continue her clinic. 'If Miss Caisse were half as humane as she claims to be, her clinic would be open today,' Mr. Kirby declared."

On June 28, the Toronto *Daily Star* reported that the Minister of Health had been visited by a delegation of 80 to 90 of Rene's patients and had agreed to join in with them to seek an interpretation of the Kirby Bill from the Attorney General.

After those meetings with Kirby, the leader of the deputation, F.F. Stevenson, wrote Rene a colorful letter telling her what it was like negotiating with the government. With refreshing insight, he described the deputation's experiences: "It seems as though the medical association have the government hog-tied. From Monday to Friday we never missed a day at Queen's Park and I thought we were getting places with Kirby and Conant until Hepburn came into the argument, and just try to get him to put anything in writing. All we could get was Kirby's statement in the press that he would frown on a Commission that would ask for a formula before they investigated the past and present treatments.

"Honestly I believe we can make them carry on the investigation your way by keeping Kirby's memory refreshed with his own statements on the subject. It is a cinch we have them worried and with the Docs hammering at them also, I doubt if the Commission is named for some time, maybe not this year. I would like to see them named right away, then we would know how they intended to carry on their investigations.

"I believe we met Hepburn on one of those days when he wasn't feeling so good, he acted like he had a bad night. Even Kirby seemed disgusted with the way he acted, as when Hepburn walked out on us, Kirby said he would get in touch with you. But still insisted he couldn't, without Hepburn's consent, give us in writing any assurance that the Commission would carry on their duties in a certain way or that you would not be fined if you did not turn over your formula, if they should ask for it before they investigated your past treatments.

"But verbally they both were very emphatic that the government would see to it that you would be fairly dealt with. Their whole argument has always been that the Bill was there and they did not have the authority to change it but they would assure us that they had no intention of letting any medical association run the government. Hepburn nearly went through the roof when I said that the Docs were all powerful.

"Again I would ask you to open your clinic and let the opposition come to you, even if you do get fined once. We can surely raise a hundred for the first one, but again I say I believe the government are ready to play ball with you. All I can ask is that you be a good Canuck and open your clinic so we can have them coming to you instead of you appealing to them. And don't let them worry you, everything is going to be O.K."

But Rene wasn't reassured. Her attitude was that the law was the law and if the government wanted her to open her clinic, they should change the law. The clinic remained closed. On July 14, the Bracebridge *Gazette* editorialized: "We predict that if some sufferer who desires Miss Caisse's aid should die while the clinic is closed, there will be a veritable roar of bitter condemnation by the general public in these parts and the target of that condemnation will not be Miss Caisse."

Two weeks later, newspapers throughout Ontario reported that Rene had finally yielded to the pleas of her patients and would reopen on August 5. She and the government had fought each other to a draw in the first round. The Kirby Bill was still the law; but the government had promised publicly not to enforce it for the time being. Both sides were now gearing up for the next round of the battle: The investigation by the newly formed Royal Cancer Commission.

CHAPTER
FOUR

I n late August, 1938, six physicians with expertise in diagnostics, surgery and radiology were named as the members of the Royal Cancer Commission. The chairman was Mr. J.G. Gillanders, an Ontario Supreme Court Justice. They were charged with investigating several different unorthodox cancer treatments in use in Canada in the late 30s, but the focus was clearly on Rene Caisse and Essiac.

For the last few months of 1938, Rene was busy treating patients at her clinic, while skirmishing with the Commission as it got underway. On October 27, she wrote them a letter declining to turn over her formula before they acknowledged the proof of her work. "I wish to know," she wrote, "whether or not I am to continue my clinic. If you wish me to close, I wish you would notify me to that effect. I do not wish to continue, if I am subject to the penalties of the Kirby Act."

The Commission declined her invitation to close her down. They didn't want to get into that routine again. Instead, Dr. B.L. Guyatt, a professor of anatomy at the University of Toronto and an early supporter of Rene's, was informally enlisted as a mediator. He had good relations on both sides.

On December 30, 1938, when the Commission was ready to begin its investigation of Rene and Essiac, Dr. Guyatt wrote Rene a long letter saying that she should be confident and cooperate fully in presenting her cases, especially those with "a pathological diagnosis and shown clinical progress with a disappearance in part or wholly of signs and symptoms."

Rene wholeheartedly took Dr. Guyatt's advice. That was what she'd really wanted to do all along, anyway: Get those doctors into her clinic and show them what she'd been doing.

When the Commission announced to the press that two of its members—Dr. W.C. Wallace of Queens University and Dr. T. H. Callahan of Toronto—would be going to Bracebridge in February, 1939, to interview Rene's patients, Rene told reporters she was "delighted with the arrangement."

Accompanied by Dr. Guyatt, the Commission members spent two days conducting the sworn—and secret—testimony of several people who had been treated by Rene. Afterwards, some of the patients told reporters that they had traveled long distances at their own expense to tell their stories under oath.

One of them, Mr. George Bruce of Hastings County, was quoted in the Toronto *Globe and Mail* as saying that he owed his life to Rene Caisse. "I came here all burned up from radium treatments. I was nothing but a withered rat, expecting to die any day. Miss Caisse treated me for six weeks, and now I am 100 percent better."

Mrs. J.C. Forsythe, of Utterston, told reporters that she testified that Miss Caisse had initially refused to treat her because she didn't have a copy of her doctor's diagnosis. "Finally Miss Caisse agreed to give me treatments. I was a cripple when I came here, and was at death's door. Now I cook for a big family, do all my own housework and all the other chores that a farm wife has to do. I owe my life to Miss Caisse."

Since the hearings were held in secret, Rene refused comment to the press, except to say she was pleased with the Commission's thoroughness and fairness. Privately she told friends that the doctors had examined some of her former patients and admitted to her—and them—that they were now free of cancer. Rene was thrilled at this latest turn of events.

But the main event was scheduled for early in March, 1939. Public hearings before the full Commission were to be held at the Royal York Hotel in Toronto. This was what Rene and her patients had been waiting for, and when it came they were ready. So many of her supporters showed up that Rene had to rent one of the hotel's ballrooms as a gathering place. Among those present were 387 former patients, from all over Canada, prepared to wait their turn to be sworn to oath and tell their stories.

The Commission wasn't interested in hearing from 387 witnesses. "She's got an army of people here," Commissioner Valin complained. Ultimately, pleading the pressures of time, the Commission allowed only 49 to testify.

The hundreds of pages of transcript of those 49 sworn witnesses is filled with heart-rending testimony. To a person they were convinced that Essiac had helped them to regain their health. Some of them told of partial and continuing recoveries when all else had failed; others described complete, almost miraculous, recoveries after they had been near death.

A man named George Mahon testified: "She helped me. If it was not for her, I would be buried." A woman named Elizabeth Stewart testified that her doctor sent her home from the hospital almost two years ago to make out her will. "It won't shorten your days," she said the doctor told her, "and it won't lengthen them."

Now, after treatment by Nurse Caisse: "I'm working every day. I milk five cows, night and morning. I'm right off the farm and have boarders and all in the house, and I have to do it all myself. I owe my life to Miss Caisse and I hope you will do something for her."

A woman named Augusta Douglas had a diagnosis by a pathologist, dated August 5, 1938: Cancer of the cervix. She was told she needed radium treatments. She told the doctor she'd rather die. "With my boots on," she said. "Thank God I had enough will power. I fought the doctors and I am still."

She recalled arriving in Bracebridge for her first treatment by Rene Caisse. "I went on a bed made in the back of the car on a mattress with a feather tick folded on it, and I could stand no jolting of the car or I would get this terrible pain in my back."

She spent six weeks flat on her back in bed in Bracebridge, having treatments. "As I lay in my bed I could see the clinic on the hill and it reminded me of the Cross on the hill of Calvary. I know you men do not care anything about this but just the same it was the only ray of hope I had in the world."

Gradually she improved. She started taking walks. After eight weeks she was able to make the 220-mile round-trip drive to Bracebridge every Saturday. She testified that her doctor told her: "If that is what she has done with a few, keep on taking her treatments. They are marvelous. They are worth a million."

Clara Thornbury weighed 72 pounds when her husband carried her into Rene's clinic. Now she weighed 107 pounds and did her own housework.

Annie Bonar's cancer spread after radium treatments. Weighing 90 pounds the night before she was to check into the hospital to have her arm—swollen to twice its natural size—amputated, she decided to see Rene Caisse instead. Four months later, she was back to her normal weight of 150 and her arm was Ok.

One witness after another told stories like that. But perhaps the most dramatic—and moving—testimony was offered, in vivid and often horrifying detail, by a woman named May Henderson.

After 30 years of chronic ill health, she was told by her doctors that her whole body was riddled with cancer. They would have to remove both her breasts and most of her insides. She wasn't up to the torture of that, she decided, and basically gave up on living.

"My eyes just looked like stones," she testified, "and I simply hadn't any life in me. I couldn't walk and by this time I was lying on the chesterfield or else on the bed most of the time. I didn't know just what was ahead of me, but someone told me about Miss Caisse."

That was in March, 1937. May Henderson went to see Rene, but Rene couldn't treat her without a written diagnosis. So May Henderson dragged herself to a doctor for another torturous examination. "He said that my condition was such that I was simply full of cancer, and that it was useless for the nurse to treat me because I would not last long anyway."

But the doctor gave May Henderson the signed paper she needed. She began the Essiac treatment. "Right away I noticed a wonderful change. I felt more steady and I slept better and I ate better, and altogether I have had about 65 treatments from the nurse. Shortly after I started with her I was able to have temporary work and I might say I never have been inconvenienced by the treatments."

Did she regard herself as cured?

"Well, pretty nearly." She explained that she still had a small lump on her right side. "It is about the size of a hen's egg, but it is softer than it used to be, and in the left side there is still some of this hard growth, but it is pretty nearly all gone."

Commissioner Valin asked if she still had lumps in her breasts.

"No," she answered. "They are completely cleared up....The breasts are quite clear now. When I first started with the nurse I looked as if I were pregnant, my body was so full of it, and it had pushed everything else out of its position, and now I think anyone would agree my figure just looks about normal. I feel as if it is normal." (In Rene's files are several friendly letters from May Henderson, dated all the way into the 1970s, and always thanking Rene and encouraging her in her good work.)

The commissioners repeatedly questioned the accuracy of the diagnoses related by the witnesses. They said that some of the doctors involved had later denied diagnosing these people as having cancer. Rene's lawyer, Edward Murphy, at one point ridiculed that argument, saying that not even the most careless doctor sent people home from the hospital with two weeks to live without being reasonably certain of his diagnosis.

Hinting at pressures on doctors to disavow their original diagnoses, Murphy said: "If this matter is done so sloppily, there should probably be a commission to investigate *that*." These people were told they had cancer, he argued, no matter what some of the doctors were now trying to say.

Near the end of the hearings, Dr. B.L. Guyatt—the anatomist from the University of Toronto—was allowed to testify about what he had seen at Rene's clinic. "I first became interested three years ago this fall," he said. "It was brought to my attention by a doctor who was a friend of mine, a prominent man."

Since then Dr. Guyatt had made periodic visits to Bracebridge. "I have not had the time or the apparatus to make a check such as I would like to have made, but I saw patients come in, in very bad shape, and the next time I went along I found improvement in a number of those cases."

That happened on at least three of his visits to the clinic, Dr.Guyatt testified. "I was so impressed that I brought the matter to the attention of Dr. Routley of the Canadian Medical Association, later asking that some investigation be made into this form of treatment. That's how impressed I was."

Continuing to follow the progress of a number of Rene's patients suffering from what he believed was cancer, Dr.Guyatt said they had definitely improved. "I would not say they are cured. I would not use that statement, because a cure of cancer means 5 years, and even then you are not sure. But certainly there has been a great benefit in those cases."

When Dr. Guyatt finished his testimony, Chairman Gillanders told Rene's lawyer that it was time to get on the record with Rene's position about revealing her formula to the Commission. "We have heard more case histories from Miss Caisse than from any other sponsor," he said. "She is the only sponsor, I think now, who has not been willing to disclose her formula."

Murphy said her position was the same as it had always been. "She would like the Commission, having heard this evidence, to pass upon it, and she will quite willingly abide by that decision."

"In other words," the chairman responded, "she is not prepared to give her formula?"

"No."

Then the chairman summarized his own position: "What she is asking us to do is to pass on the case histories she has given us, without the Board having any knowledge of what the substance contains, or the theory of its operation or administration."

"Exactly," Murphy said.

After a long debate between Murphy and the commissioners about Rene's refusal to reveal the formula, Commissioner Valin said: "You are seriously, I think, prejudicial to your cause in not revealing the formula. We may be favorably impressed. We don't know. As far as we have gone, we cannot tell. There may be something in it, as Dr. Guyatt says. He thinks it is something which should be investigated further. That is what he suggested, to have some independent investigator go ahead, and he appeals to the Ontario Medical Society to have it investigated.

"That is his impression, and he is a disinterested party. He is not biased. We feel we should like to pursue our observations further, and that is the reason why we want the formula."

Then the chairman said: "I think Mr. Murphy knows the attitude of the Commission."

"Yes, I do," Murphy said.

"We will advise you when the next meeting is to be held," the chairman said.

"That is the best thing to be done," Murphy responded.

"It is understood we are through hearing Miss Caisse's cases?" Commissioner Young asked.

"Oh, yes, that is closed," Murphy said.

"Definitely," the chairman agreed. And with that, the testimony of Rene's witnesses was concluded.

A few weeks later, near the end of March, came the testimony from the other side, the doctors. A Dr. Richards and Dr. R.T. Noble, the registrar of the College of Physicians and Surgeons, presented signed documents from several doctors saying that former patients of theirs had not benefited from Rene Caisse's treatments and had since died.

Rene was present as Dr. Richards and Dr. Noble damned her with all the evidence they could find. One of her patients who had died was named William Allen. After listening to the doctors proclaim that Mr. Allen had not benefited from Essiac, Rene responded: "Mr. Allen came to me with a tube in his bladder, and in a very bad condition, and they had no hope for him at all. A great number of these cases are hopeless cases, who came to me perhaps for treatment, and I tell the family—I did not tell the patient—but I tell the family that it is hopeless, and I cannot hope to do anything other than possibly give them comfort. If they care to take a few treatments they do so, and if they go away and die, then these records go against me."

Commissioner Valin challenged Rene: "Apparently you say you cannot cure an advanced case."

"No, I did not say that. If the organs are destroyed, yes. I cannot build new bodies."

Dr. Richards introduced as evidence the August 10, 1937, death of a man named Richard Patterson. Rene responded: "His doctor gave him three days to live when I took him, and he lived a year and a half."

At one point, Dr. Richards stated that some of Rene's patients who survived had been previously treated with radium, which was the source of the cure. "In other words," Rene shot back, "if the patient lives, you take the credit for radium, but if the patient dies, radium has nothing to do with it."

Dr. Richards produced the case of one of his former patients who had ceased radium treatments in favor of Rene's clinic and later died. Rene's answer to his accusation was: "She was dying when she came to me. She weighed about 83 pounds. She had been burned deeply with radium. You could hear her breathing through a big hole in her chest, to the bone, and when she breathed, a whistling came through the outside, and she was given up by Dr. Richards. They could not give her any more radium.

"She had no other treatment, and I took her out of pity, and she lived for two or three years, in fair comfort. The burn healed, and she gained weight. I think she weighed about 118 pounds. She was fairly comfortable, to the end, and I feel quite proud of my treatment."

A few of the reports from physicians actually admitted that their former patients claimed to have received benefit from Essiac, most notably pain relief. Even in this hostile accumulation of reports, the theme of pain relief was heard again. But in these post-mortem reports from doctors, it was usually mentioned briefly and in passing, as if a patient's relief of pain was not the point; the point was discrediting Rene Caisse.

It was a brutal experience for Rene, listening to these doctors lay waste to any notion of possible benefit coming out of Essiac. Finally she said to the commissioners: "Dr. Noble and Dr. Richards are both bringing up a lot of patients whom I took through pity's sake. They are not taking up my proven cases, which have benefited. A great number of these patients came for one or two treatments, and never came back, and I could not save them. I did not want to take them at all, because I knew the cases were hopeless. Every case was given up by the medical profession before I even took it."

At the end of this stage of the Commission hearings, the commissioners once again asked Rene for her formula. Once again, she told them that she did not want the formula taken from her and immediately shelved as worthless. "I want to know that suffering humanity will benefit by it. When I can be given that assurance, I am willing to disclose my formula, but I have got to know that it is going to get to suffering humanity."

Chairman Gillanders said he wouldn't admit any merit before receiving the formula. Rene said they didn't have to admit it publicly; just admit it privately. "I feel that I am entitled to your decision on the merits of it, before I give it."

"In other words," Gillanders said, "you are not prepared now to give the Commission the formula?"

"No, I am not."

"You will, however, submit whatever comments you have on this evidence?"

"Yes, I will be very glad to do that."

Rene did later respond in detail to the charges that many of her patients had since died. But the overall burden of the hearings had taken a heavy toll on her—physically, emotionally and financially.

She had taken her fight as far as any one person with such limited financial resources could have taken it. Amid publicity and pressure, the Canadian parliament had been forced to debate about Essiac—and had come within three votes of legalizing it.

She had mobilized what Commissioner Valin complained of as "an army of people" to rally support. And now that the battle appeared to be winding down, her exhaustion and despair—even bitterness—was apparent in a powerful letter that she fired off to Premier Hepburn on April 19, 1939, a few weeks after the testimony of Dr. Noble and Dr. Richards.

"I have submitted a large number of histories of cancer patients to them," she wrote. "They then demanded cases pathologically proven, where no other treatment had been used. I was just able to present two of these cases cured, as the majority of my cases have tried everything Medical Science has to offer before coming to me. I have many proven cases cured who have had other treatment before coming to me.

"Dr. Richards maintains that though long periods have elapsed between the time of the radium treatments and my treatments (even though recurrences have appeared) that the radium is still working on them and is responsible for the cure, but if the patient dies, radium has nothing to do with it.

"Now they are demanding that I give an account of every patient I have been unfortunate enough to lose. Not taking into consideration the fact that these patients are dying before they ever come to me and are given up by the medical profession as hopeless. I am trying to do this to the best of my ability, but one might just as well ask a doctor why one operation is successful

and another one fatal. He will say that the case was too far advanced or that the patient had a weak heart. This is the answer
I will be compelled to give in some cases.

"The Committee that came to my clinic, on examining my
patients, did not hesitate to tell patients that they were cured,
patients that I was still treating. They seemed perfectly satisfied,
even enthusiastic, over what they saw. I gave them the pathological proof of one case that had not been treated elsewhere, and is
absolutely clear of cancer.

"I gave a copy of this pathological proof to the court stenog-
rapher to give copies to each one of the Royal Cancer Commission, and at the last sitting of the committee none of them had
copies of this pathological report, and Dr. Callahan did not
remember seeing it. I have since sent registered copies to the
secretary of two such cases.

"Now, I do not mind trying to comply with their request. It
is putting me to a lot of expense which I cannot afford, for though
I am accused in some of the letters Dr. Noble presented against
me of taking all the money I could get from people, I have had
so little given me that it has been a great struggle to carry on. I
asked for a report of the last meeting and they charged me fifty-
seven dollars for it. When I tell you that my bank account is not
one hundred dollars, you will understand why it is difficult for
me to supply all the material the Royal Cancer Commission are
asking for, and keep my clinic going.

"I am considering seriously closing, God knows I have done
my best for these cancer sufferers, but if you had heard Dr. Noble
and Dr. Richards pull my work to pieces you would believe me
to be a criminal. I had an operation eight weeks ago for bursitis
on my arm, which instead of helping me, made my condition
worse, and the surgeons cannot account for that. I have had to

work at my clinic with my arm in a sling, spending the rest of my time in bed trying to get back the use of my right arm.

"If you can in any way shorten this investigation, I will appreciate it very much. I feel they have enough material to make a decision one way or the other. I have gotten beyond the stage where I care which way they decide. If you could read the testimonials sent to Dr. Noble by members of the profession, their denial of their own diagnoses, and their suggestions on how to convict me of illegal practice, you would see that they have no intention of being fair. If Dr. Richards had to give an account of the number of patients who die under radium and deep X-ray treatments he would have work to do for the rest of his life.

"Dr. Noble put in a list of patients who signed a petition to you in 1937, with two hundred and ten names of patients who claimed to have benefited by my treatment. He handed this to the Royal Cancer Commission saying that most of these were dead. There are thirty-two of these dead, one of these was killed in an automobile accident, several went back for radium treatment when I closed my clinic last May, two had amputations after leaving me and died, one hundred and seventy-eight are living. I do not think this is a bad percentage.

"I am sorry to trouble you about this, but I am going down to see Dr. Lewis today, and with my arm in the condition it is, I may be ordered to bed for an indefinite period and I want you to know that I have complied with every demand of the Royal Cancer Commission."

But the Commission's investigations dragged on for months. Rene kept her clinic open, but she was dogged with problems and feeling as though she was being left hanging, not knowing what was coming. On November 2, 1939, she finally made a plea directly to the Minister of Health, Harold Kirby. "I am writing to ask if there isn't some way that you can speed up the report from the Royal Cancer Commission on my cancer discovery," she wrote to him. "It seems to me that they have had ample time to decide for or against my treatment. I have put before them more evidence than any other sponsor. They admitted this in my presence at the last meeting on July 4th. If they have decided against it I have other plans and am anxious that they should make their decision one way or the other.

"The doctors have in a body refused to give any diagnosis of a case coming to me. I have people visiting my clinic begging for treatment and as you know I cannot take them without their doctor's diagnosis. Would it be possible for you to give me permission to treat any patient who came to me stating that his or her doctor told them that they had cancer, and to have them sign a statement to that effect? I would appreciate your opinion on this matter."

In December, 1939, the Commission delivered its Interim Report to parliament. Limiting itself to ruling on the cases of the people who had testified in support of Rene and Essiac, the Commission dismissed several of the diagnoses of cancer as incorrect— or had letters from doctors disavowing the diagnosis. Other cases were ruled cured by previous treatments with radium or X-ray.

"In the 49 cases presented there were only 4 in which the diagnosis was accepted and in which recovery occurred apparently from Miss Caisse's treatment," the report stated. But even in those four cases, the report went on, the Commission later received signed statements calling into question the validity of the cure. In one, for instance, the report stated: "The Commission now has a signed statement from the surgeon to the effect that the growth he removed was not cancer."

It was a tortuously written report designed to deny any credit at all to Rene and Essiac. Implicit in it—though not stated—was that all 49 witnesses were somehow mistaken about their own cases. The report implied that "out of this large practice" of Rene's, only these 49 people stepped forward—completely ignoring the fact that another 338 people waiting in the ballroom were denied the opportunity to testify.

The report concluded: "After a careful examination of all the evidence submitted, and analysed herewith, and not forgetting the fact that the patients, or a number of them, who came before the Commission felt that they had been benefited by the treatment which they received, the Commission is of the opinion that the evidence adduced does not justify any favourable conclusion as to the merits of 'Essiac' as a remedy for cancer, and would so report."

Having dismissed Rene and Essiac, the Commission made one final attempt to persuade her to turn over the formula. In the last paragraph, the report said: "If, however, Miss Caisse is desirous of having her treatment further investigated, and wishes to submit thereon further evidence, and is prepared to furnish the Commission with the formula of 'Essiac,' together with samples thereof, the Commission will be glad to make such investigation, in such manner as is deemed desirable and warranted."

From the beginning, the commissioners had often said that they only wanted to investigate remedies that might hold some promise. They were physicians themselves and they didn't mind saying on the record that they had better things to do with their time—and the Commission's budget—than to pursue worthless remedies.

And yet, at the end, in the paragraph after they tried to write off Essiac for once and for all, there it was again: We want the formula. But why? The contradiction would seem to be readily apparent.

On January 11, 1940, after the report had been approved in parliament, it was released to the Canadian press, which gave it heavy coverage. It was front page news. One newspaper quoted Rene: "The Commission would not consider any recovery due to Essiac unless there had been no other treatment previously taken. I have been obliged to treat so many cases sent to me by doctors after everything in medical science had been used ineffectively. I have not been allowed to take a cancer case without a doctor's diagnosis, and in the majority of cases, a doctor will not give me a diagnosis unless he considers the patient beyond the help of medical science."

Four days later Rene wrote an angry letter to Premier Hepburn. "I received a copy of the Royal Cancer Commission's report on my work. In spite of the fact that they slashed my evidence, I am still the only one of the eighteen applicants who has so much as one cure to their credit. They admit four cures, but they say that in two of these cases they have received sworn statements from the doctors denying their own diagnosis. I think I am entitled to copies of these sworn statements, and I would appreciate it very much if you will personally see that I get them."

She concluded: "For the sake of suffering humanity, I am begging you to support my work and again put my bill before the Legislature."

Hepburn let Rene's request go by. Two months later, Rene wrote a long letter to one of the local newspapers detailing her criticisms of the Commission's report. The letter filled almost one full page of the newspaper, showing how the Commission had belittled the results she had accomplished.

In the case of a man named Peter Hanon, for instance, who had testified for Rene, the Commission concluded that an accurate diagnosis would have been "spastic colon," not cancer. After outlining his case at length, Rene concluded: "He was sent home to die and in such a bad condition and the end was so near that he was advised to go to a hospital where he would require special medical care. Nothing could be done for him.

"I succeeded in stopping the hemorrhaging, his evacuation became normal, the pain ceased, he increased in weight and is now a healthy man."

The newspaper accompanied Rene's letter with a full page editorial supporting Rene's arguments and mentioning all the area residents who knew with certainty from personal experience that Rene's treatment worked. "Scores of patients volunteered their evidence," the editorial said. "Insistence was made that Miss Caisse disclose her formula. Her refusal to do so was apparently based on the belief that if she did so, the finding would be that it was valueless and then later on the medical profession would discover a treatment for cancer that would be very much like hers. In this way she would lose the credit for all her work and effort and her patients would not be benefited. The report of the Commission on cancer seems to justify the fear that appeared to be in Miss Caisse's mind."

And with that farewell, Rene Caisse pretty much disappeared from public view—and public controversy—for almost 20 years. She was now 52 years old. She had fought a battle, lived through turmoil—treating desperately ill people one day, sitting in a roomful of doctors listening to them savage her work the next day—that would have worn down the strongest human being. The Kirby Bill was in force and with the Commission's ruling that Essiac had no merit, there was reason to believe that the government might begin enforcing it against Rene. Nonetheless she kept her clinic open for the time being. She continued to treat patients. A year after the Cancer Commission report, May Henderson dropped her a short note to say that the Essiac still "has magic in it for me."

On January 19, 1940, Dr. R.A. White, in a "Dear Madam" note to Rene, wrote: "For your own information and if it is of interest to you, Mrs. Otto Latondress has been suffering from a Squamous celled Carcinoma of the Cervix for about the past year. Yours truly."

(Fifteen months later, Otto Latondress swore an affidavit stating that after his wife's treatments by Dr. White, "she weighed ninety-four pounds, and could hardly walk." After forty treatments by Rene Caisse, his wife was fine. "She was examined by Dr. White last Friday, and he found that there was no trace of cancer.")

On April 3, 1940, a few months after war broke out when Hitler invaded Poland, Rene wrote an interesting letter to the general manager of Parke Davis, a huge American pharmaceutical corporation.

She wrote: "I have a solution that I use effectively to stop hemorrhaging and have been using this as long as I have been treating cancer. It was brought to my notice how valuable this would be in time of war to treat the soldiers. It will stop any bleeding almost instantly. I have affidavits from many patients to this effect, and if you will read the enclosed circular you will notice that Dr. B.L. Guyatt specially mentions this in regard to my treatment. I wonder if your company would be interested in this, and if you could suggest any way that this could be made available for use in the hospitals overseas, first aid stations, soldiers' kits, etc.

"I never thought of this as a separate discovery; it was just a part of my treatment of cancer cases, but now I feel that I should make every effort to make this available to all those who need it."

Rene still wanted to help people in any way that she could. During her political battles of the 1930s, she hadn't boasted of, or even claimed, any special solution she had developed to stop hemorrhaging. To her, it was just part of the treatment. But with World War II being fought, her first instinct was that this might have value to wounded soldiers—and she wanted them to have it.

It was a touching gesture. But apparently Parke Davis ignored it. There is no record of any response, and Rene never said that she received one. So any value her solution might have had to those wounded soldiers was lost forever.

At the same time that she was volunteering her help to the war effort, she was being threatened with arrest for violating the Kirby Act. It was becoming nearly impossible for her to get written diagnoses from doctors, and finally Rene gave up.

In 1942, paranoid about being imprisoned and, as she later described it, "in a state bordering on collapse," she officially, and permanently, closed her clinic and left Bracebridge. She moved—or more accurately, retreated—to live quietly in North Bay.

It was the end of that era of her life. A vastly different one was about to begin and almost certainly the farthest thing from Rene Caisse's mind was that the new era would end with her—and her work with Essiac—once again back in the news.

CHAPTER
FIVE

I know very little about Rene Caisse's life from 1942 until 1959.

Sometime probably during the 1930s, she had married. Her husband's name was Charles McGaughey. He was a barrister, then a district magistrate, then a juvenile court judge. From the few newspaper accounts about his career, he seems to have been a widely respected member of the community. There are a few pieces of correspondence between Mr. Mc-Gaughey and the Canadian government, indicating that he supported Rene's activities and was prepared to write strong letters on her behalf when he felt she was wronged.

The old newspaper photographs of Mr. McGaughey show a handsome man with a full head of hair and a nice smile, holding a pipe and wearing a three-piece suit. He and Rene didn't have any children, but he had four by a previous marriage.

Mr. McGaughey was from North Bay, which probably influenced him and Rene to move back there when they decided to leave Bracebridge. Sometime after they moved, Rene apparently suffered what she herself later described as a nervous breakdown. After what she'd been through, it's not hard to understand why. The breakdown, I've heard, didn't last long. One of Rene's best friends told me that Rene didn't even check herself into a hospital for treatment. She just stayed at home and did whatever she did until she recovered.

That's the sum total of what I know about Rene's breakdown. Even her friends don't seem to know much about that chapter of Rene's life. For all practical purposes, she just disappeared for a few years. I wish I knew more. But I don't. One of the eeriest sensations I experienced in researching her story was near the end of reading through her files.

Rene kept everything that dealt with Essiac, and also with cancer. Thousands of pages of correspondence, newspaper clippings, doctors' diagnoses—seemingly every shred of paper dealing with cancer—and when those files came to me, they came in large suitcases, all the papers and all the years thrown in together.

After I had spent days reading and organizing this massive history Rene kept, it suddenly dawned on me that from 1942 until 1959 there was almost not a single sheet of paper. No letters, no newspapers. Nothing. It sent chills up my spine. To this day, I don't know if she kept files for those years and they were misplaced, or if there was never a file.

In an ironic twist, the last sheet of paper before the 17 year gap in her files, dated January 9, 1942, is a letter from the chief of the Proprietary or Patent Medicine Division of the Canadian department of Pensions and National Health.

Addressed to Rene at her North Bay address, it states in its entirety: "Dear Sir: Enclosed you will find license authorizing sale of the following preparation under THE PROPRIETARY OR PATENT MEDICINE ACT for the calendar year 1942: R.M.C. Kidney Pills, Reg. No. 20027. Please forward copies of labels, wrappers and all other literature used in connection with the above-named product."

After all the sweat and blood and tears she lived through to treat cancer patients with Essiac, at the moment she was retreating into her own private life, the government sent her a "Dear Sir" letter issuing her a patent for...kidney pills. I didn't know whether to laugh or cry.

But I had heard about those kidney pills in Bracebridge. They were sold in the drugstore. Rene gave them out. People said they helped. Some of the locals still remember them. I don't know what was in them, or what they did, but in the middle of all her life and death battles over the treatment of cancer, Rene somehow managed to develop kidney pills—and get a patent on them.

Rene herself, as far as I've been able to find out, didn't write much or speak out much on the pills. She knew they were effective and she used them. But she seemed to take it for granted, and they weren't a part of any crusade. Her attitude was as if to say, doesn't everybody develop patentable kidney pills in their spare time?

What Rene did with the patent, what happened with the formula for those kidney pills, I have no idea. I haven't been able to find much information about the pills—except that some people in Bracebridge remember the drug store selling them many years ago—after that 1942 letter from the Canadian government.

In 1943, Rene's husband Charles McGaughey died of pneumonia at the age of 57. Rene's best friend told me that Rene took his death very hard. Despite her paranoia about arrest, she had very quietly and very privately—only her closest friends knew anything about it—continued to treat certain desperately ill cancer patients with Essiac.

The hours were long, she was apparently away from home traveling when necessary to treat people, and the secrecy created stress. When her husband died of complications from the pneumonia, Rene blamed herself. Her friend told me that Rene felt guilty for not devoting herself to nursing her husband's illness. Torn between her patients and her husband, she felt she had failed her husband.

According to her friend, Rene became even more reclusive after her husband's death. Many old friends and patients didn't see her at all for years. But it is known that she traveled a lot. She took frequent trips—especially during the winters—to Florida, where she stayed with a sister.

Another sister was married to a wealthy man in the state of Washington, and Rene apparently visited them as often as possible. What little portrait of Rene I have in those years is one of a lonely woman, restless and searching, and alienated from any hope of ever seeing the world recognize and appreciate what she had accomplished with Essiac. Listening to her old friends—and her own statements made later—I got a strong sense that she had reconciled herself to a tragic defeat. It had to be a very painful reconciliation.

Sometime in the late 1940s or early 1950s, Rene moved back home to Bracebridge. She was in her 60s by then, and still badly overweight. At that stage of her life, and after what she'd been through, it would have been easy to slip into complete retirement and give up altogether.

But Rene remained active. "Now, like Grandma Moses, I paint pictures," she wrote. From all accounts, she was a prolific artist, who loved to spend hours doing her oil paintings of nature—flowers, countrysides—and still life of all kinds. The paintings are quite lovely. Not the work of a professional artist; but a talented and skilled amateur.

She gave the paintings away, to friends and family members. There are people all around the Bracebridge area who are quick to pull out a Rene Caisse painting and show it proudly to a visitor.

She passed some of her time writing about cancer and Essiac. She was a good writer, with an intimate knowledge of disease and medicine, based on a lifetime of medical experience. Everything she had learned and witnessed after treating thousands of cancer patients convinced her that cancer is a systemic disease, not a localized one, spread through the body via the blood stream, and that surgery, radium or X-rays targeted specifically at the area of a tumor is attacking the symptom and not the cause.

In other words, a healthy system purified by healthy blood will not sustain a cancerous tumor. In a diseased system, if the tumor is surgically removed or destroyed with radium or X-rays, the cancer will eventually reappear elsewhere if the system isn't cleaned out and purified. Some of the herbs in Essiac, she wrote many times, acted as blood purifiers, attacking the cause of cancer rather than the symptoms.

In one of her essays, written sometime during the 1950s, Rene wrote: "There are those of us who feel that cancer is more than a local disturbance in some distant organ of the body. This was impressed on me very deeply when, after making the rounds of a cancer ward in one of our best treatment centers, the surgeon in charge said to me: 'This is not the answer.'"

By the late 1950s—with the same prescience as Rachel Carson who won international fame for her book, *Silent Spring*—Rene wrote in her personal essays a warning about agricultural pesticides and food preservatives, about all the chemicals we were spraying into our environment. Five years before scientific fear of Strontium 90 in radioactive fallout persuaded President Kennedy to sign the treaty against atmospheric testing of nuclear weapons, Rene was writing essays warning of the dangers we were facing from nuclear testing.

But no one who knew her ever accused Rene Caisse of being all business, of having no time for play. All her old friends are quick to mention her sense of humor. She used to say it was the only thing that kept her sane and allowed her to survive all the heartbreak she lived through.

Her friends say that to some degree, she was a romantic at heart. They say that she liked men, loved to joke with them, do a little harmless flirting with them, all her life. In her younger years, she wrote some beautiful love poems. Later she wrote a sweet, charming poem about younger women. For the wry glimpse it provides into how Rene saw the personal side of ordinary life, here is her poem entitled "An Honest Fact":

The men of to-day
We regret much to say
Do not respect the ladies
In the good old-fashioned way.
The girls of to-day
Do not demand respect they say
They encourage the man
In a very wrong way.
They study "vamp" glances
And do "toddle" dances
Nor wait for the men
To make the advances.
Oh! Girls of today
'Tis a very wrong way.
If you want your whole life
To be happy and gay
Create a modest style
And a good old-fashioned smile.
It is surely up to you
To wear blushes that are true
Then you'll find, the gentlemen
Will show respect for you.

In 1958, Rene was 70 years old. In addition to her writing and painting, she was still whipping up meals and holding court in her living room with nephews and nieces and old friends. They all say that she was remarkably energetic for a woman of her years and weight.

And though the walls around her use of Essiac were high, indeed—very few people were allowed to know what, if anything, she was doing with it—she was still treating some unknown number of cancer patients.

After a gap of almost 17 years in her files, one of the first papers from this later era of her life is dated September 10, 1958. It is a letter to the new Premier of Ontario, Leslie Frost, and it is a stern protest against recent governmental threats made to Rene. "Some time ago I wrote a letter to you," she wrote, "asking if it would be possible to put my Bill before the legislature in order to legalize my 'Essiac' treatment of cancer.

"You replied, saying that you had sent my letter on to the Cancer Commission. Well, they sent an officer here to arrest me but when I explained to him what I was doing for sick people, he did not arrest me but ordered me not to treat my patients. He told me to write to the College of Physicians and Surgeons and ask for an interview with Dr. McPhedran, which I did and was shocked to get such a rude reply."

After 25 years, the government was still sending people to arrest Rene and she was still talking them out of it. Rene closed her letter to the premier: "The patients who were improving under my treatments are frantic and come begging for treatment. It is the hardest thing I have ever had to do, to turn them away. Is there anything that can be done to remedy this situation? I would appreciate a reply."

Premier Frost replied that Rene should get in touch directly with the Deputy Minister of Health, Dr. W.G. Brown. In October, 1958, Rene wrote Dr. Brown a long letter, outlining her position and saying, in part: "I had a man, a Mr. Schwartz, from Oshawa, call on me last Sunday. He said that since I treated him eight years ago for cancer of the spine, he has been, and is now, in perfect health.

"I have a case now, a woman from North Bay with cancer of the breast, with secondaries under the arm. She was losing the use of her arm. Now it is localized in the breast, and she can use her arm quite freely, and has no pain. The primary is beginning to reduce. She is frantic because I have been ordered to stop treating.

"I am glad that when Dr. McPhedran sent his policemen here to arrest me, that I had not too many patients to turn away. I closed my clinic years ago, but patients came begging for treatment at my home, and I could not turn them away. Now the onus is on the medical profession. I *have* to turn them away. Do not feel sorry for *me*, Dr. Brown; feel sorry for the many who cannot have the benefit of this Essiac treatment for cancer."

In January, 1959, Dr. Matthew B. Dymond, the Minister of Health—and a doctor who would in the future play a critical role in the story of Rene Caisse and Essiac—assured the Bracebridge representative to parliament that the College of Physicians and Surgeons would not prosecute Rene without notifying the Minister or his Deputy. "I gathered," Dr. Dymond wrote, "that it is their hope that Miss Caisse's activities might be controlled by means of surveillance, and that no prosecution would ever be necessary."

So I do know that Rene remained active—and combative when necessary—even in those reclusive years from 1942 until 1959 when she stayed out of the spotlight as much as possible—and the letter from Dr. Dymond indicates that her fears about the government spying on her were not merely paranoia. The government was spying on her.

But at the age of 70, her life was about to change dramatically again. After years of living quietly and without attention from the outside world, she was going to be under close scrutiny, with lots of questions being asked, and serious medical people paying close attention to Rene Caisse and Essiac.

CHAPTER
SIX

I n February, 1959, a Canadian named Roland Davidson visited the New York City office of Ralph Daigh, the Editorial Director and Vice President of Fawcett Publications. Fawcett published magazines—including the most popular men's adventure magazine of the era, *True Magazine*—and paperback books. It was a prominent American publishing company.

That meeting led to Rene Caisse's return to public life, at the age of 70.

Ralph Daigh later wrote a 33-page, typewritten private memo about the events that began with that meeting. One of the most fascinating documents of the whole Rene Caisse story, Daigh's memo describes—in sometimes chilling detail—what happened the day he met Gordon Davidson and what followed in Daigh's own personal search for the truth about Essiac.

Daigh wrote that Gordon Davidson was a complete stranger who showed up at his office urging *True Magazine* to publish a story about this nurse in Canada who had been treating and curing cancer patients for more than 30 years. Davidson himself had been treated by the nurse for a severe case of ulcerated hemorrhoids and believed that he had been cured.

Davidson had with him a large envelope filled with documents. "Mr. Davidson stated," Daigh wrote in his memo, "that in his opinion the material in the envelope could be used to produce the most important story ever published by *True*, The Man's Magazine. It was Mr. Davidson's rather naive opinion that a detailed story of Nurse Caisse's thirty-five years' experience in allegedly curing cancer, alleviating and eliminating pain for cancer patients, would bring her the world-wide acknowledgment to which he felt she is entitled."

As a veteran editor, sophisticated in the ways of politics and the media, Daigh understood how naive Davidson was to believe that one magazine article could accomplish anything like that. It was going to take a lot more than a magazine article to win medical acclaim for Rene Caisse.

As it turned out, the documents in Davidson's envelope weighed more than ten pounds. At first glance, Daigh wrote, they were "a great hodge podge of newspaper clippings, personal correspondence, case histories of persons suffering from various forms of claimed malignancies." Daigh approached them "with the skepticism that any editor might be expected to exhibit in connection with the efficacy of a so-called cancer cure."

Daigh spent four or five hours studying the material. There were case histories of 120 patients. "Very few of these cases were properly validated with pathological reports from laboratories, but some were," Daigh wrote. "In addition to claims of curing these malignancies, the case history reports very frequently mentioned that severe pains suffered by these people were almost without exception alleviated by Nurse Caisse's remedy."

There it was again, the theme of pain relief associated with Essiac. Since this was Daigh's first exposure to the subject, he had no way of knowing how common that theme had been. "In many of the instances," he wrote, "the pain was reported alleviated after only one, two or very few treatments."

A few of the case histories reported cures for illnesses other than cancer, including stomach ulcers, goiter, hemorrhoids and subsequent bowel stoppage. The package of documents contained the early petition signed by physicians, Dr. Emma Carson's testimonial to what she had seen at the clinic, Dr. B.L. Guyatt's endorsement, Rene's correspondence with Premier Hepburn and with many of her patients, as well as the newspaper accounts of the parliamentary battles of 1938 and 1939.

After reading the material, Daigh took it to the Editor of *True*, Douglas Kennedy, and discussed it with him in detail. Taking himself out of the story and writing in third-person, a common journalistic practice, here is how Daigh described that conversation:

"Both editors thought that indications were present supporting the assumption that Essiac was a substance of importance to the medical world and to humanity. Both editors were impressed by the repeated assurance that patients were taken off narcotics shortly after treatment with Essiac started, and found no necessity for further use of narcotics. Both editors were impressed also by the numerous evidences of proof that skin cancer had been eliminated in many patients, and that such cures were subject to visible proof."

But Daigh and Kennedy—as responsible editors—reluctantly agreed that no story could be written without new proof based "on additional patients under absolute clinical and pathological conditions. It was obvious from the material inspected that Nurse Caisse had treated many thousands of patients in a rather helter skelter manner and had been more interested in curing suffering humanity than in establishing pathological proof that cancer existed, although there was some pathological evidence in the names of many doctors who had allegedly certified malignancy in the patients treated."

Just as reluctantly, Daigh and Kennedy concluded that *True Magazine* did not have the time or the money it would take to conduct such studies. *True* was, after all, a magazine, not a medical research institution. They decided they would have to return the material without writing a story.

In early March, 1959, Daigh sent back the package with a note saying that it would be impossible for Fawcett to conduct such "a long and expensive re-evaluation."

But Daigh couldn't shake off his doubts. He found himself "plagued with the possibility that this nurse in a remote section of Canada might have a remedy for which the whole world was looking."

Later in March, he requested the material back. He studied it again, carefully, and reached the conclusion that he would be "derelict as an editor and a member of the human race" if he didn't do all he could to find out the truth about Essiac.

He contacted a friend, Paul Murphy, at the Science Research Institute and asked him to read the documents and give an opinion. "After a week," Daigh wrote in his memo, "Mr. Murphy returned, convinced by the possibility that Essiac, if not a complete cure for cancer, was at least a palliative, and impressed, too, with the possibility that even though the remedy might not be as efficient against cancer as claimed, an examination by the proper medical authorities and scientific personnel, with laboratory testing, might prove Essiac beneficial as a remedy in the area of ulcers, goiter, hemorrhoids or skin lesions."

Daigh decided to take Paul Murphy with him to Bracebridge to conduct "an on the ground examination" and interview Rene Caisse before making any decisions. He called Rene and arranged an appointment.

In early April, 1959, Daigh and Murphy arrived at Rene's home. "Nurse Caisse was found to be a most personable woman in her late 60s," Daigh wrote in his memo. "A devout Roman Catholic and possessed of the calm assurance and patient good humor characteristic of a superior individual."

Their first interview with Rene lasted seven hours. She told them her story, going all the way back to the fateful day in the early 1920s when she encountered the woman patient with the badly scarred breast.

After hearing Rene's account of her political struggles in the 1930s, Daigh concluded that the College of Physicians and Surgeons had become "stiff-necked" in their demands for her formula, but that Rene probably hadn't understood how to wage the kind of public relations campaign that would have won the College's cooperation.

In a touching passage that helps to explain Rene's withdrawal from the world after the 1939 Cancer Commission Report, Daigh quoted her describing how she'd felt: "This was the end. I had fought so long, and I was tired, and I was older. I felt I had done everything in my power to assure giving my remedy to the public, and I couldn't do any more."

Daigh quoted Rene explaining her belief about how Essiac worked: "Occasionally nature makes an error in cell construction, and when this cell attempts to fit into the pattern to which it is assigned, it is repelled by the healthy cells with a violence only nature is capable of producing.

"The natural tendency of the normal cells is to throw out, destroy or consume the unnatural cell, and if the body is strong enough, this fact is accomplished.

"If, however, the abnormal cell is strong enough to get a foothold in the human body, and the normal cells cannot throw it out or surround it and thus inhibit it, the cells in that particular area go wild and the body destroys itself in that area with a cancerous growth.

"My remedy, in some way I do not understand and am unable to explain, strengthens the natural defense mechanisms of the body and enables the normal cells to destroy the abnormal cell as nature might expect a strong body to do.

"There also seems a possibility that my preparation weakens abnormal cells, because I am able to observe sloughing off of great masses of diseased tissue from cancer of the breast, cancer of the rectum or even internal cancer.

"I am forced to look upon Essiac as a great tonic and giver of strength to the body so that nature is aided in removing the abnormalities of growth which are defined as stomach ulcers, goiter, hemorrhoids—and cancer."

At the end of their seven-hour interview, Daigh told Rene that he and Paul Murphy planned to do more investigation. If they concluded in favor of Essiac, they would invite her to the United States to work with a reputable medical center.

Rene said that would interest her, but she was reluctant to take up residence in a strange city at her age. She didn't want to leave her brother. He was not well and she was taking care of him. And she didn't want to indulge, Daigh wrote, "in the opening of an old war which she had already dismissed as lost."

But Daigh had learned that three of the doctors who had signed her petitions many years earlier were still alive and living in Bracebridge. He told Rene that he would like to interview them before he left town.

Early the next morning, a Sunday, Daigh and Murphy went looking for the doctors. What they found shocked them both and persuaded Daigh that there was more of a mystery here than he'd realized.

The first doctor they located was Dr. A.F. Bastedo—the physician who had persuaded the Bracebridge City Council in 1935 to turn over to Rene the old British Lion Hotel.

"Dr. Bastedo proved extremely uncooperative, and even rude," Daigh wrote in his memo. "When informed that Mr. Daigh and Mr. Murphy would like to ask him a few questions about Nurse Caisse, his reply was: 'I will not discuss her in any manner.'"

When Daigh persisted and said that he had come a long distance to find out what he could, Bastedo said: "You will get no help from me or any other doctor, I don't think."

"With that he walked from the porch of his home, turning his back," Daigh wrote, "to a garage where he kept his car, across the street, and apparently drove off to church."

Then Daigh and Murphy tracked down Dr. E. G. Ellis. Daigh described him: "In his late 70s, a very handsome and distinguished looking individual, who lives in a small house on the main street of Bracebridge, and is still practicing. Dr. Ellis was planting sweet peas when we approached. He graciously invited us into his house."

But when they explained why they were there, Dr. Ellis seemed disturbed. Even though he finally consented to answer their questions, "it was obvious that he was using an extreme economy of words, although he was at all times studiously courteous."

They asked Dr. Ellis if he had ever signed a petition for Rene Caisse. He denied that he had. Daigh was carrying the original in his briefcase. He chose not to confront the doctor with it. He wanted to keep the conversation going.

They asked Dr. Ellis if he had ever sent cancer patients to Rene Caisse. He denied that he had. Daigh had the case histories in his briefcase revealing "that a number of patients were sent from

Dr. Ellis or with Dr. Ellis' permission to Rene Caisse." Daigh said nothing about it.

"As the discussion continued," Daigh wrote in his memo, "Dr. Ellis intimated very strongly it was not a good thing for a doctor in Canada to discuss Nurse Caisse in any way, and it would certainly be very bad for any doctor who admitted any faith in her treatment or admitted sending her patients.

"Dr. Ellis' attitude in this respect reminded us of Nurse Caisse's statement, that doctors had been forbidden to treat patients treated by Nurse Caisse after 1939 or 1940, and had been forbidden to discuss her or her work."

In one of the most chilling passages in all the documents that exist about Rene Caisse, Daigh described at length what happened next:

In answer to a direct question, Dr. Ellis would not deny that the situation was as Nurse Caisse stated.

Dr. Ellis stated flatly that he knew of no cases of cancer that had been cured by Nurse Caisse.

Neither did he know of any cases of goiter, stomach ulcers or hemorrhoids that had been cured by Nurse Caisse.

Thereupon Mr. Daigh asked Dr. Ellis the following three-part question:

1. Do you think that Nurse Caisse is a charlatan, a fraud?

Dr. Ellis' answer: "No."

2. Do you think Nurse Caisse was only after money?

Dr. Ellis' answer: "No, I don't think she made very much money."

3. Now, Dr. Ellis, you have stated that you do not believe Nurse Caisse is a charlatan or a fraud and that you do not believe she was motivated only for mercenary reasons. If I understand your answers correctly, it would seem to me that the only possible definition left for Miss Caisse is that she is a psychotic. Do you believe this to be true?

Answer by Dr. Ellis: "No, she is not a psychotic. She is a sincere, well-balanced person."

Dr. Ellis was probed for other definitions of Nurse Caisse that would shed light on her operation as a practitioner offering a cure for cancer, and Dr. Ellis' answers were always reserved and courteous. He was completely unwilling to condemn her as a person, or in connection with the administration of her treatment.

Thereupon Mr. Murphy asked the following question: "In view of the efforts being made by medicine today to find an effective treatment or cure for cancer, do you think Nurse Caisse's preparation and treatment should be evaluated scientifically and clinically to determine whether or not there is any merit to the remedy?"

Dr. Ellis paused briefly, and then an emphatic "Yes."

The third doctor Daigh and Murphy interviewed was Dr. F.M. Grieg. Daigh described Dr. Grieg in his memo as "a bachelor in his late 70s and for many years one of the leading doctors in the community."

Greeting them at his front door, Dr. Grieg "evidenced extreme reluctance to discuss Nurse Caisse or her remedy," Daigh wrote. They had to persuade Dr. Grieg to invite them into his living room.

"In the beginning his attitude was somewhat antagonistic, but as the meeting progressed, he became more cordial and finally he answered questions freely, although tersely."

Dr. Grieg denied much knowledge of Rene Caisse's activities and refused to admit that he had ever sent her patients or signed a petition in her behalf—although Daigh had proof of both in his briefcase. Once again, Daigh chose not to confront the doctor with the evidence.

Grieg denied any knowledge of cancer cases cured or in any way helped by Rene Caisse. "He somewhat surprisingly admitted, however, that he knew of a case of stomach ulcers that had been cured by Nurse Caisse," Daigh wrote. "This was a man Dr. Grieg admitted had been his patient."

Daigh asked the doctor what he regarded as a cure in this case?

The doctor replied: "The man couldn't keep anything in his stomach. He lost weight. He had severe ulcer pains. He couldn't sleep. After a few treatments from Nurse Caisse, the pains disappeared, and he was able to eat anything. I kept track of him for a number of years, and there was never any reappearance of the trouble. I am certain he had ulcers."

Immediately following this admission, Dr. Grieg "resentfully attempted to end the interview," Daigh wrote.

Daigh asked a few quick questions before leaving:

Is it not healthy for doctors in Canada to discuss Nurse Caisse?

Grieg refused to answer the question.

Is Nurse Caisse a charlatan or a fraud?

"No."

Was she only after money?

"I don't know how much she made. She used to take a little black bag to the bank every week, but she didn't make a regular charge and I understand the contributions weren't very large. If she had been after money, she would have charged."

Is Nurse Caisse a psychotic?

"No."

If she isn't any of the above, what is she?

"She was a well-intentioned woman, who thought she had a cure."

But if she didn't have a cure and still persisted in using it over the years, doesn't it follow that she is a charlatan, after money, or psychotic?

"No, she is a good woman. She is not mentally unbalanced, and she certainly wasn't out to take anyone's money. She may have done some good for some people, but I don't know about it."

Should a qualified laboratory investigate Essiac?

"I think it would be a good thing to test it once and for all," Dr. Grieg replied.

The reactions of the local doctors were enough to persuade Daigh and Murphy to ask Rene Caisse to come to the U.S. to make a scientific evaluation of Essiac. But when they returned to her home, she greeted them by saying: "I'm rather sorry that you have come back."

She told them that she had decided against going, although the challenge was intriguing. Her brother needed her. She had had a heart attack a few years ago and her health was not good. She was overweight and afraid that starting all over in a strange city would be too hard on her.

But Daigh was ready for Rene's reluctance. Before traveling to Bracebridge, he had prepared a formal agreement—just in case. He read it aloud to her: She would be guaranteed all expenses in Boston to use Essiac on humans with cancer and animals inoculated with cancer. All tests and experiments would be under the direction of Dr. Charles Brusch at the Brusch Medical Center in Cambridge, Mass.

Dr. Charles Brusch was—and still is—a respected physician. In 1955, he administered the first polio vaccine in Cambridge. For many years, John F. Kennedy was one of his patients—and friends. Dr. Brusch was one of the physicians who treated Kennedy for Addison's disease. Kennedy laid the cornerstone to Dr. Brusch's medical clinic.

Among Dr. Brusch's other patients have been many of the most prominent names in Massachusetts, including former House Speaker John McCormack and his wife. The Brusch Medical Center was—and still is—one of the largest medical clinics in the state.

Daigh told Rene that the agreement included the stipulation that if the tests proved satisfactory to Dr. Brusch, then a corporation would be formed and a means found for commercially developing and marketing Essiac.

After she had heard the entire agreement, Rene Caisse said that this was exactly what she had wanted for more than thirty years. It was an emotional moment for all of them. She said she would go to Cambridge.

They signed the agreement. Rene arrived at the Brusch Medical Center on May 22, 1959. And thus began one of the most exciting and hopeful periods of her life—at the age of 70.

CHAPTER SEVEN

I n May, 1959, Rene flew to Boston and was met by Ralph Daigh. She was given a comfortable apartment in the Commander Hotel in Cambridge, not far from the Brusch Medical Center. At the clinic, three rooms—a waiting room, a dispensary and a treatment room—were made available for Rene's use. Her treatments were to be supervised by Dr. Brusch's director of research, Dr. Charles McClure. Dr. McClure would personally maintain the case history files.

One of the first patients treated was a 40 year old woman named Lena Burcell. Four years after surgery to remove a cancerous breast, the cancer had reoccurred in her lung. X-rays showed her to be terminally ill.

She received her first treatment from Rene Caisse on May 26, 1959. Almost immediately, her ability to breathe improved markedly. Prior to treatment with Essiac, Mrs. Burcell had complained of severe joint pains. These pains lessened noticeably, she told the doctors. She lived for three months.

Exploratory surgery—followed by biopsy—on a 37-year-old man named John Cronin confirmed that he was terminally ill with inoperable cancer of the right lung. An alcoholic, Cronin was known as a difficult and unreliable patient.

When he started treatments with Rene Caisse, he was too weak to climb one flight of stairs comfortably. He was suffering severe pains in the area of his chest incision and was being given narcotic painkillers.

Cronin had seven weekly treatments, each consisting of one ounce of Essiac orally and one ounce by intramuscular injection. He told doctors that the pain in his chest had disappeared, and he was not as short of breath. He could climb several flights of stairs without discomfort and had taken up his old hobby of swimming.

A drinking binge landed him in the V.A. Hospital, where he was threatened with loss of his veteran's medical benefits if he continued non-V.A. treatment. When he got out of the V.A. hospital, Cronin went back to the Brusch Medical Center saying he would gladly sacrifice his veteran's medical care in favor of the relief he was receiving from Essiac.

The file merely notes that under the circumstances, no further treatment was given by Rene Caisse.

A 58-year-old man named Wilbur Dymond was suffering from prostate cancer. After two months of treatments, all hardness in the prostate had vanished, except for one small nodule. He reported to doctors that he no longer suffered excruciating pain during urination.

Russell McCassey was suffering from a basal cell carcinoma of the right cheek, proven by biopsy. The open lesion had been present for months. He had not had X-ray or radiation treatments. After four treatments—both orally and intramuscular injections—in two weeks, the color of the lesion changed from red to pale pink. The lesion reduced in size. The central ulcer crater was disappearing.

After three more weeks of treatments, the lesion was healed, leaving only a small white mark where the biopsy incision was made. The file notes that this case appeared to be cured.

Those are typical examples. The supervisor, Dr. McClure, wrote about his experiences with Rene and Essiac: "After having personally observed Miss Caisse administer her remedy for cancer on known cases of malignancy for about three months, and the results of such administration, I am certain the remedy is efficacious. It is to be regretted that the patient sample is so small, although small as the sample was, her gratifying results on all cases are indisputable.

"The sense of well-being engendered in the patients is heartening and easily noticed. The return of strength and will to do, obvious. The relief from pain is possibly the most dramatic change. In those cases of cutaneous cancer the evidence of quick healing and regeneration visible and positive."

To supplement her treatment of patients, Rene agreed—at Dr. Brusch's urging—to perform experiments on mice inoculated with human cancer. Initially the Memorial Sloan-Kettering Institute in New York agreed to provide the mice.

The first group of mice treated with Essiac was returned to Sloan-Kettering in mid-June, 1959. According to Dr. Brusch's records, Dr. Philip C. Merker of Sloan-Kettering called to say that Sloan-Kettering was very interested in what it was seeing: namely, a physiological change in the cancer growth characterized as "a tendency of the cancer cells to amalgamate and localize."

But then Sloan-Kettering said that it would have to have the formula in order to continue any further studies. Dr. Brusch and others seriously considered that possibility, but Rene remained adamant that she would not release the formula until she had some guarantee that it would not be "bottled up in the laboratory" or permanently shelved as worthless.

It was the same old Catch-22: Admit its merit and I'll release the formula; we can't admit merit until we know what's in it. The experiments would have to continue without the cooperation of Sloan-Kettering.

A prominent Boston surgeon who was familiar with the work being done at the Brusch Medical Center suggested that the National Cancer Institute might be helpful in future animal experimentation. Ralph Daigh contacted the NCI. They were interested, but placed the same demand as Sloan-Kettering: the formula first.

So the experiments on mice continued without the involvement of the huge cancer research centers. Here is what Dr. Charles McClure and Dr. Charles Brusch later wrote of those experiments: "On mice it (Essiac) has been shown to cause a decided recession of the mass, and a definite change in cell formation."

On the treatments of patients, their final report concluded: "Clinically, on patients suffering from pathologically proven cancer, it reduces pain and causes a recession in the growth; patients have gained weight and shown an improvement in their general health.

"This, after only three months' tests and the proof Miss Caisse has to show of the many patients she has benefited in the past 25 years, has convinced the doctors at the Brusch Medical Center that Essiac has merit in the treatment of cancer. The doctors do not say that Essiac is a cure, but they do say it is of benefit. It is non-toxic, and is administered both orally and by intramuscular injection."

During the time Rene spent at the Brusch Medical Center, Dr. Charles McClure mailed questionnaires to some of Rene's former patients. He received back several testimonials from people

treated as long as 31 years earlier, including some who had testified for Rene at the 1939 Royal Cancer Commission hearings:

Clara Thornbury—treated 22 years previously. Alive and well
at 75. (She eventually died in 1975 at the age of 91.)

Nellie McVittie—treated 23 years previously. Alive and well
and still in touch with Rene in 1959.

Wilson Hammell—treated 31 years previously.

Eliza Veitch—treated in 1938. Age 76 in 1959.

After about a year, with only a limited number of patients
available for treatment—due to American Medical Association
restrictions on remedies of unknown substances—and
laboratories increasingly reluctant to supply mice inoculated with
human cancer, Rene returned home to Bracebridge. She was convinced that the labs were under pressure to stop cooperating with
her. Once again, she was pessimistic about Essiac ever gaining
recognition and acceptance.

But she had made a friend and believer out of Dr. Charles
Brusch. They remained on good terms, in communication and
cooperating with each other about the future of Essiac for the
rest of Rene's life. To this day, as I write this, almost 30 years
after Rene's work in Cambridge, Dr. Brusch remains an outspoken advocate of Essiac as a valuable treatment for cancer
patients.

CHAPTER
EIGHT

s the 1960s began, Rene remained active. She was supplying Essiac to Dr. Brusch. She was secretly treating patients out of her home in Bracebridge. But now she was also trying to interest large institutions in the idea of exploring Essiac's capabilities.

In March, 1960, she wrote to the Biochemical Institute at the University of Texas, telling them what she had. She received back a polite note, dated March 22, 1960, from a Research Scientist named Alfred Taylor: "We are interested in checking various plant products for their effects on cancer growth from the standpoint of laboratory tests with animals bearing cancers....We are always glad to check materials which can be used in our testing programs."

But nothing came of it. She tried to interest Merck & Co., the huge pharmaceutical manufacturer. Merck's Office of General Counsel responded in legalese saying basically that they would have to have the formula, and then they would make up their own minds in their own way in their own time. It was not a response designed to encourage Rene to put her hopes in them— or to indicate that they knew of or had any interest in this opportunity to get to the truth about Essiac.

A physician in Arcadia, California came to believe in Essiac. In October, 1960, he wrote a long letter to Rene offering his strategy for a new crusade for Essiac: Find a "few trusted physicians" to run "pilot studies." Then offer the results of these new pilot studies to the profession. "It seems advantageous to offer the results of a new testing program which has not already been assigned a 'thumbs down' position by a legislative body," he wrote. And then they should present "an improved, tested chemotherapy called Essiac."

But he counseled great patience. The testing program "would take a minimum of one and one fourth years before the date of product availability. This may be much too short a time because of the nature of the disease. The diagnosis of a Cure is arbitrarily based on a five year period."

There was a lot of wishful thinking of that sort going on all through the 1960s. But there wasn't the organization or the money or the political clout to bring any of it together into a major political movement or to persuade the big institutions to negotiate a research arrangement with Rene. And with Rene well into her 70s by now, she was no longer strong enough to fight the same kind of publicized political fight she had waged three decades earlier.

Essiac remained alive through word of mouth. People from all over North America found Rene when they needed it. She'd get phone calls in the middle of the night from people in Europe who wanted to get some. In her spare time, Rene produced a pamphlet: "I was Canada's Cancer Nurse." She wrote more warnings about our food and our environment. In one, she railed against poisoned additives, chemical processing of flours, oils and fats, and chemical aging of such foods as cheese.

She urged people to take four steps:

"1. Do NOT eat these foods if alternatives are available.

2. Urge our governments to take action against these conditions.

3. Read the labels (especially the small print) on everything you buy to eat or drink.

4. Patronize the manufacturers who produce foods without added colors and other additives, and who are growing foods in soil not contaminated with chemicals and where they do not use poisonous sprays."

Even now some of her former patients from as far back as the 1930s stayed in touch with her, offering encouragements. May Henderson, who had testified so powerfully at the Royal Cancer Commission hearings in 1939, was still alive and well and corresponding with Rene.

In 1971, when President Richard Nixon declared his "War On Cancer," May Henderson wrote to Rene: "I guess you read the headlines in our papers recently. 'Nixon prepared to spend billions to find a cure.' I guess that and the fact that a dear old friend had to undergo surgery and have a breast removed recently has kept me wondering what is going on—if anything—with your wonderful work and formula."

May Henderson noted that she was now 75 years old and experiencing "usually good health." A year later she sent a copy of Rene's "I Was Canada's Cancer Nurse" brochure to her Member of Parliament, asking him to get involved in a new crusade. She received back a polite thanks, but no thanks note.

In 1973, when she was 85 years old, Rene decided to make one last try with the medical establishment. She contacted Sloan-Kettering and asked them if they wanted to renew the encouraging tests they had done in 1959. Dr. Chester Stock, a vice president and associate director for administrative and academic affairs, said they would be willing to run tests on mice if Rene would send them some Essiac.

Rene agreed. Sloan-Kettering was interested in tumor regression, so she began supplying them with one of the Essiac herbs. In her experiments with mice at the Christie Street Hospital in Toronto in the early 1930s, she had determined that this was the herb that caused the regressions. (The others acted as blood purifiers.) She gave Sloan-Kettering detailed instructions on how to prepare the herb as an injectible solution.

It will probably never be known outside of Sloan-Kettering what actually happened in their experiments with the Essiac herb. But the tests do seem to have gone on for an extended period and there is at least one piece of documentary evidence that Sloan-Kettering was getting some positive results.

On June 10, 1975, on the letterhead of the Sloan-Kettering Institute for Cancer Research in Rye, New York, Dr. Chester Stock wrote to Rene: "Enclosed are test data in two experiments indicating some regressions in sarcoma 180 of mice treated with Essiac. With these results we will wish to test enough more that I should ask if you can send more material. If you have questions about the data, please don't hestitate to ask them."

"Two experiments indicating some regressions in sarcoma 180 of mice treated with Essiac." That one sentence alone written by a top Sloan-Kettering official in 1975 should be cause for even the most skeptical to agree that Essiac should be taken seriously by today's medical and scientific communities. (Sarcoma 180, incidentally, is a type of cancerous tumor often used in medical research.)

But unfortunately—despite those encouraging test results in 1975—the Sloan-Kettering tests came to a halt the next year. Other test results were coming out negative, so Rene looked into the situation. On August 22, 1975, Dr. Stock wrote her: "I will check to determine whether our laboratory group is not adequately informed on making up the Essiac from the material you supplied. I will see that the next test is above reproach."

But when Rene received an explanation of how Sloan-Kettering was preparing the injectible solution, she was horrified. They
had ignored her instructions. They weren't boiling the herb.
They were freezing it, then thawing it. As far as she was concerned, they were making one mistake after another. In an angry
scrawl, she wrote on Sloan-Kettering's explanation: "All wrong.
Rene M. Caisse."

Her reaction was cold fury. She terminated the agreement with
Sloan-Kettering and stopped providing them with the material.
(Two years later, in 1978, a group in Detroit filed a class action
suit against the U.S. government, seeking to legalize the importation of Essiac for cancer treatment. In his sworn affidavit in
that case, Dr. Stock stated: "We have tested Essiac in a very
limited way against sarcoma 180 in the mouse. We have not seen
any consistent activity." But he admitted: "After our testing was
done we were informed that we should have had two prepara-
tions for test and also that we made improperly the injection solution from the dried material supplied to us. We were never
provided full information about the nature of Essiac.")

But even with Sloan-Kettering out of the picture and Rene almost 90 years old, Rene and Essiac were about to burst, once
again, into the public spotlight.

CHAPTER
NINE

I n 1977, the editors of *Homemaker's*, a nationally distributed Canadian magazine based in Toronto, heard an awesome story: An 88-year-old nurse from Bracebridge had been successfully treating terminally ill cancer patients for 50 years with her secret herbal formula.

By its own account, the magazine assigned a team of very skeptical reporters to investigate. What those reporters discovered over the next six months caused a profound transformation in their attitude.

In the Summer, 1977 issue of *Homemaker's*, the magazine reported: "Essentially, Rene's story was true. She had been getting remarkable results against many kinds of cancer with Essiac, and she had been prevented from carrying on treatment unless she revealed the formula. Whether it would have been swept under the rug by a jealous medical hierarchy, as she feared, or hailed by a grateful profession that heaped honors at her door, is a question that no one can answer, since Essiac never stood the test of controlled clinical studies."

Until the last moment, the editor of *Homemaker's* wrote, the staff had "real reservations about publishing a story that would give false hope to cancer patients. The knowledge that our

decision would possibly cause traffic jams in Bracebridge as the
public beat a pathway to an old lady's door didn't help, either.
But the consequences of the alternative—not to publish—were
too ghastly to contemplate. There were too many 'ifs.' What if
Essiac works? Even if Essiac only relieves suffering, it must be
tested. Clearly, the possibility for good far outweighed the nega-
tives."

The editor mentioned their initial skepticism about Essiac and
wrote that the staff members had asked each other when it had
crumbled. "When asked this question individually, we all had the
same answer. Shearer (the magazine's executive vice president)
was the last person I queried: 'It was the day I realized that if I
was told I had cancer, I would visit Rene. It wouldn't be the only
thing I'd do. Hell, I'd try anything—the works, conventional and
otherwise—but I'd go see Rene first.' That's a pretty strong indication of our feelings."

The *Homemaker's* article then outlined at great length the entire saga of Rene Caisse and Essiac, going all the way back to the
day in the 1920s when Rene was told by the old woman with the
scarred breast about the Indian who gave her the herbal formula
that cured her breast cancer.

The article described the political battle of the 1930s "that
reached right to the floor of the Ontario legislature, and made
headlines all over the continent."

Rene was vividly described by the journalists who had come
to know her: "Though Rene was wary, extremely sensitive to
doubt, and frightened that at any moment 'they' (the arm of the
medical profession that she felt had squelched her in the past)
would stifle or subvert us, she had a brilliantly sharp mind and
almost total recall of names, events and personalities.

"Each time we visited her over the next few months, she would
be sitting in her favorite easy chair, resplendent in a vivid

flowered dress, the winter sun glinting off masses of costume jewelry, her hair hidden under a jaunty sable wig. She was always ready to produce more documents, newspaper clippings, letters from supportive doctors, and case histories as well as before-and-after photographs of cancer patients plucked from drawers or cardboard boxes stashed under her bed. And when we allayed her suspicions by setting up her own tape recorder as backup, she talked into our recorder about her experiences. She had lived many years with the possibility of fines and arrest hanging over her, and trust did not come easily.

"She resented our insistence on the need to verify every fact. Insomniac, discouraged and impatient, she often expressed the fear that she would not live to see Essiac recognized. In modest circumstances, she seemed genuinely disinterested in reaping any financial rewards, and was determined that Essiac should never fall into hands that would exploit it for unseemly profit."

The *Homemaker's* reporters wrote of interviews they conducted with some of Rene's former patients who had testified at the Royal Cancer Commission hearings in 1939 and were still alive in 1977.

One of the witnesses in 1939 was a railroad engine watchman named Tony Baziuk. His lip cancer was so severe that it disfigured his whole face and forced him to give up his job. Six months after he started Essiac treatments, he was working again and could, as he told *Homemaker's* almost 40 years later: "Eat for one man, work for three, and sleep like a little baby."

The magazine quoted May Henderson at 81 reminiscing about Rene's clinic in the 1930s: "We liked to get an early start," Mrs. Henderson told *Homemaker's*, "because the clinic was always filled. We tried to get our treatment before lunch, have a bite to eat in Bracebridge, and then drive back. It only took a minute to get the injection and drink the tea, and the patients used to exchange progress reports while we waited."

May Henderson said that she was still healthy in 1977 and had never suffered any recurrence of her cancer.

The *Homemaker's* reporters interviewed Dr. Chester Stock at Sloan-Kettering. He claimed that their tests with Essiac were not encouraging, but he "doesn't rule out the possibility that Essiac could be effective against human cancer."

About their interview with Dr. Stock, *Homemaker's* reported: "The material Rene sent him was 25 years old, and only one herb—the injectable one—was used on the mice. Rene never did send him either the complete formula or all the materials."

According to *Homemaker's*, Dr. Stock told them that he would agree to conduct further tests if Rene would give him the formula for Essiac so that Sloan-Kettering could administer both the injections and the oral treatment.

Attempting to play the role of mediator, *Homemaker's* passed that offer on to Rene. "Her refusal was instantaneous, and failed to yield over the next weeks in spite of our urging. She felt it was futile to go on testing on animal cancer; she wanted Essiac used on patients, or at the very least, on human cancer in animals. Furthermore, she did not believe that Sloan-Kettering would prepare the material properly.

"'Last time, they froze it,' she claimed. 'They might as well have been injecting distilled water.'"

The magazine also talked to Dr. Charles Brusch. He praised Essiac and told them about his recent treatment of a man named Patrick McGrail for cancer of the esophagus with herbs supplied by Rene Caisse.

The article went to press only 14 weeks after McGrail's treatment with Essiac began. McGrail was reported to have gained 11 pounds and was "feeling a heck of a lot better." (When Dr. Brusch chose McGrail as an example, he had no way of knowing that McGrail would still be alive and well ten years later.)

At the end of their research, the management of *Homemaker's* believed enough in what they had learned that they made an official proposal to Rene. As it was described in the magazine: "In the hope that we might speed Essiac on its way through the bureaucratic maze with no more loss of time, we offered to set up a trust to represent her in any dealings she might have with the government, Cancer Institute or any interested pharmaceutical companies."

Much to their disappointment, Rene turned them down. At the end of their story, *Homemaker's* concluded: "There's a tragic and shameful irony in the Essiac tale. In the beginning, a simple herbal recipe was freely shared by an Indian who understood that the blessings of the Creator belong to all.

"In the hands of more sophisticated (and allegedly more 'civilized') healers, it was made the focus of an ugly struggle for ownership and power.

"Perhaps our cure for cancer lies back in the past, with our discarded humility and innocence. Perhaps the Indians will some day revive an old man's wisdom, and share it once again. Perhaps this story will be the catalyst; if so, our efforts will not have been in vain."

The *Homemaker's* article caused an immediate sensation in the Canadian media. Newspapers picked up the story. Television crews arrived in Bracebridge—one of them to prepare an hour-long documentary about Rene and the history of Essiac that was later aired on Canadian television.

Rene Caisse's two phones were ringing practically around the clock. People besieged her home, pleading for treatment. She received threats from people saying they would take action if she didn't turn the formula over to them. She finally had to unlist her phone and—for a while—accept police protection.

Rene received a flood of letters after the article appeared. "My husband, Yves, has been doing just wonderfully well, with your blessed Essiac," one woman wrote. "Your formula has been a miracle for Yves and God willing—we so want him to continue with it."

"I thought of you many times over the years," a woman named Annie Goynt wrote. "I hope you remember me. I came to you for treatment thirty years ago and I have seen many pass away with cancer and always thought of you and what a shame you could do nothing. But at last from what I have read in the paper and an exclusive report in the *Homemaker's* Magazine your cure has at long last been accepted. I only hope it is used as it should be used."

"We read of your treatment 'Essiac' in the *Homemaker's* Magazine," another woman wrote. "I would like to tell you how pleased we are with the progress of my brother who has been on your treatment for a few weeks."

The Essiac was acquired with the help of their family physician, she wrote. "There was improvement from the start. Now, about 8 weeks later he is certainly much better." He had gone from too weak to do anything for himself to driving his own car and looking after his show horses. "His case was considered terminal with only a short time to carry on. Please accept our thanks and wishes for continued recognition of this great discovery and also for better health for you."

One physician from Coldwater, Ontario had the courage to write to Rene saying that one of his patients had improved over the last three weeks on Essiac. "Both appetite and strength are better," he wrote under his official letterhead. "She is anxious to get home and is being discharged from the hospital on Monday. Thanks once again for your help."

Rene wasn't surprised. She took all the fuss in stride, and even continued to treat certain patients who were able by one means or another to work their way through all the defenses she had built up around herself.

But the most significant breakthrough of Rene's defenses—perhaps in her whole life—was made by Dr. David Fingard. A handsome and well-dressed man of about 70 who could really turn on the charm when he wanted to, Fingard was a vice president of the Resperin Corporation, a Canadian company that had interests in the pharmaceutical field.

Resperin had physicians on its board of directors, including Dr. Matthew Dymond, who had once been the Ontario Minister of Health—the official Rene had complained to about government harassment in the late 1950s. Fingard himself was a research chemist who was credited with involvement in the discovery of a drug that was effective in treating tuberculosis.

After reading the *Homemaker's* article, Dr. Fingard met with Rene and did his own research and came out of it wildly enthusiastic about Essiac. He shared that enthusiasm with Rene.

Finally, in the fall of 1977, Rene was persuaded to turn over to Resperin the formula for Essiac. Her contract with Resperin granted her $1.00 upon signing, and $250 a week for the six months Resperin agreed to conduct tests of Essiac.

At 89, Rene had tired of battling the medical establishment. She believed that Resperin was big enough and powerful enough to prove Essiac's legitimacy.

Once again the story was alive in the Canadian press. Resperin's top executives began giving enthusiastic interviews. After the Canadian Federal Department of Health and Welfare approved Resperin's plan to test Essiac on humans, Dr. P. B. Rynard—the Resperin chairman and a Canadian M.P.—was quoted in one newspaper as saying: "They looked carefully at all the facts and reviewed case histories which were very helpful. And one thing they discovered is that it wasn't toxic in any way....There is no doubt that it (Essiac) is effective for some types of cancer."

David Fingard went so far as to tell one reporter that Essiac was "one of the greatest discoveries in modern science." He told the Orillia *Journal*: "We have found certified cases of cancer ranging over a period of 25 to 30 years which have been cured by Essiac." He quoted the 1975 memo from Dr. Chester Stock at Sloan-Kettering saying that they had seen regressions in tumors in mice.

On November 25, 1977, the Ottowa *Journal* reported on two cancer patients who said they were feeling better after treatment with Essiac. Their doctors claimed there was no improvement in the condition of their tumors. But one of the patients—a 22-year-old Toronto *Star* employee who was not identified, at her request—was suffering from cancer in her pelvic bone that had spread to her lungs. She was quoted: "I received radiation and chemotherapy, and I swore I would die before I would go back for any more chemotherapy. I'm taking Essiac now and I feel all right. I come and go just as any normal person and do a day's work."

The paper also quoted a surgeon named Dr. John Barker who said he hadn't seen evidence of tumor regression in patients using Essiac. But their appetites had improved and they experienced less pain. In Dr. Barker's own words: "It's quite possible that there is something in the Essiac formula which stimulates appetite and decreases nausea and also relieves pain."

There it was again: The theme of Essiac as a pain reliever in cancer patients. Spoken over several decades, by patients and doctors alike. In 1978, it looked at long last as though Essiac were finally going to receive the controlled scientific scrutiny it had so long deserved.

In the spring there were several newspaper stories reporting that Resperin, with the approval of the Federal Department of Health and Welfare in Ottowa, was launching its tests of Essiac on human cancer patients. Resperin's chairman, Dr. P.B. Rynard, cautioned readers that it would be some time before the results would be known. "The complexity involved in a study of this kind is mind-boggling," he said.

Resperin left no doubt about their own optimism. One of the physicians working with Resperin, Dr. H.D. Wilson, was quoted as saying: "We know it's going to be scientifically proven by the best minds in the country."

But somehow Resperin's study went awry. Within months, Rene Caisse complained publicly: "I think I was able to accomplish more myself." She charged Resperin with carelessness in their studies. Resperin denied that, but the study dragged on.

On August 11, 1978, Rene Caisse celebrated her 90th birthday. The Mayor of Bracebridge, Jim Lang, an old friend of Rene's, personally organized a party for her. Friends and former patients came—some of them by the bus load—from all over Canada and the U.S. to share the day with Rene.

One newspaper reporter described the scene as the guests arrived: "They lined up to greet the guest of honor, who sat beaming in an easy chair. Miss Caisse is short, somewhat overweight, and looks years younger than her age. Her faculties are very much intact. She instantly recognized patients she hadn't seen for 35 years—and remembered their names."

There were speeches. Rene spent the day laughing and crying as she listened to the heartfelt tributes from men and women who credited her with literally saving their lives, some of them more than forty years earlier. The newspaper reporter wrote: "Scores of those present told the Muskoka *Free Press* that their only claim to life had been the administration of Essiac, when all other treatments had failed."

A couple of months after her birthday party, Rene was asleep in her den when the phone rang in her bedroom. In a hurry to reach the phone, she slipped and fell and broke her hip.

In excruciating pain, she managed to drag herself to the phone and call her old friend Mary McPherson. Even in that moment she didn't lose her sense of humor. She made a smart crack at her own expense about how clumsy she was and asked Mary to please hurry over.

When she arrived, Mary couldn't get in. Rene had the screen door latched shut from inside. Mary could hear Rene moaning in pain. The ambulance arrived and the attendants had to tear the screen door off its hinges.

Rene was so heavy that they had a terrible time lifting her onto a stretcher and negotiating their way through the house and out the door. They took Rene all the way to a hospital in Toronto for surgery. Some days after the operation on her hip, Rene was brought home. But her friends say that the medication had left her weak and groggy and that she was never herself again. She died on December 26, 1978, at the age of 90.

She was buried in a cemetery near Bracebridge. Several hundred people attended her funeral on a cold day in the snow. At her memorial service, they listened quietly as Father James Grennan eulogized Rene as a person who "manifested love and concern for humanity," and who wanted only to "further the well-being and health of her fellow man."

He added: "History may have further to say about her work someday."

CHAPTER
TEN

I don't know all the details of what happened with the tests by the Resperin Corporation. But what was initially supposed to be a six-month study dragged on for a few years. As late as 1981, David Fingard was quoted in the Kitchener-Waterloo *Record* as saying, "Speaking loosely, we already have evidence of (Essiac) cures, but the evidence is not sufficient to convince the scientific world. But we are getting excellent results."

That same newspaper story announced that the results of the government-approved test were expected to be released shortly. "Fingard says he is confident that Essiac does cure, or at least control, cancer in patients, depending on how early in the diagnosis it is given," the newspaper reported. "He also has confidence in it as a preventive. He and his wife have been taking weekly two-ounce doses (twice as much as usually recommended) for the past two years."

An accompanying article told the story of a cancer patient, Murray Braun of Kitchener, who was convinced that "he is alive and well today because he refused conventional follow-up cancer treatment three years ago in favor of Essiac, an Indian herbal remedy."

After surgery for testicle cancer in 1978, tests revealed "cancer markers" in Braun's blood. He was told at Princess Margaret Hospital in Toronto that he would have to have four weeks of radiation treatments. "If I had gone through all that, could you imagine what would be left of me now?" Braun told the newspaper. "I'd probably be dead by now."

Instead he got accepted into the Essiac test program. After ten days of Essiac, he said, the color returned to his face. After three weeks, the warmth returned to his body. "On Essiac I started feeling really good," Braun said. So good that he took up skiing again.

But despite cases like Murray Braun, in 1982 the Canadian government shut down Resperin's tests, calling them "flawed," and accusing Resperin of poor quality control in its experiments. The director of the Canadian Health and Welfare Department's bureau of prescription drugs admitted that there was no concern about Essiac's safety. It was safe, all right. But he was quoted as saying that they "cannot say this is an effective treatment."

Patients who were already using Essiac would be allowed to continue using it, in the government's words, "purely on humanitarian grounds." On those same grounds, future patients who could fight their way through the bureaucracy might also be allowed to use Essiac legally.

On December 8, 1982, a man named Ed Zalesky of Surrey, B.C., one of the cancer patients who had been treated with Essiac provided by Resperin, expressed his outrage at all the obstacles placed in the way of people who needed Essiac. In a letter to the editor of an Orillia newspaper, he wrote: "My life expectancy in 1977 was from six months to two years maximum. The fact that I'm 'clean' (according to our over-worked staff at the Vancouver cancer clinic) and still very much alive I owe in great part to Essiac. I was fortunate enough to be one of the people involved in an Essiac test program conducted by Resperin Corporation."

He went on: "I had a terrible time convincing my doctor to submit the short reports required by Resperin to compile test results, let alone to make any commitments. It seems that many doctors refuse to complete the forms, or conveniently 'forget' or make them so vague as to be useless.

"That Essiac gives relief from suffering in many cases and prolongs life there is no doubt. Why can't the people who administer the cancer funds give it a fair trial? It isn't going to hurt anyone. The medical profession should stop playing 'God' and allow us cancer patients to use the treatment of our choice."

He concluded: "I am now three years past my final death sentence, well, working full time and then some, and enjoying life, thanks to this 'unproven' compound." (Ed Zalesky was still alive and well five years later in 1987.)

When the government was criticizing Resperin's tests, David Fingard told the press that Resperin could even sell Essiac as an herbal tea if they didn't make any claims for its curative powers. But Resperin, he said, wanted Essiac to be officially accepted as a cure. "We don't want to sell it as a tea through stores," he was quoted as saying. "The only way we want to sell it is as a cure."

Resperin didn't give up after the government shut down their tests—and apparently Sloan-Kettering remained interested. On May 12, 1983, David Fingard sent a telegram to Dr. Charles Young at Sloan-Kettering, thanking him "for your interest in ascertaining the possibility of Essiac curing cancer. We naturally feel optimistic based on present results. Also delighted with your offer to come to Toronto for a meeting."

Five months later, on October 5, 1983, E. Bruce Hendrick, the chief of neurosurgery at The University of Toronto's Hospital For Sick Children, wrote his letter to the Canadian Minister of Health—quoted as the epigraph to this book—saying that Essiac appeared to have benefited children under his care sufficiently to warrant serious scientific testing.

Once again, after the latest round of controversy over Essiac, this time sparked by the *Homemaker's* article in 1977, the authorities did everything in their power to discredit and dismiss Essiac—and yet Essiac just would not disappear and die. Cancer patients continued to speak out in its support. Some physicians who had worked with it were willing to risk censure to push for more research.

That's been the story of Essiac for more than sixty years now, ever since those eight physicians signed that first petition to the Canadian government in the 1920s. Rene Caisse could never have dreamed when those first doctors showed up at her front door to arrest her, and then refused to do it after they heard what she had to say, that she had just experienced the perfect metaphor for the next sixty years of Essiac.

And so the battle continues. In my case, I had never even heard of Essiac until 1985. When I did first hear of it, I certainly wasn't looking to commit my life to an uphill struggle, any more than Rene Caisse was when she casually asked that woman what had happened to her breast.

In 1985, I was devoting all my attention to my thriving chiropractic practice in Los Angeles, where I treat a large roster of patients who include some of the most successful professional athletes in the world. Among my patients are track stars, world-class weight lifters, both men and women, and members of NFL teams.

Previously I had spent five years developing a new technique that offers my patients important benefits in the healing of injured muscles and the relief of pain. I was contracted, for instance, by the Baptist Hospital in Nashville, Tennessee, one of the largest orthopedic hospitals in southern America, to instruct them in how to implement that technique into the programs of their pain control unit.

I was—and am—proud of that work, and happy to be helping people to heal themselves. I feel that I am a success in my chosen career, respected in my field, with a long list of present and former patients who will vouch for my integrity and sincerity in anything I undertake.

One day in 1985 a friend of mine introduced me to a woman who was striking in how private she was about herself.

My memories of this woman are fresh. Certain phrases and words remain indelibly with me, along with her tones and expressions. She gave the impression of great fragility. Small and raw-boned, she had obviously lost weight. Her appearance was one of delicate survival, a balance between life and disappearance from life.

As we got to know each other and she came to trust me and respond to my curiosity, she began to tell me the story of Rene Caisse and Essiac. She had met Rene many years earlier when she had gone to Rene for treatment of her cancer. She had been in remission ever since. She regarded it as a miracle.

She and Rene had become close friends. She told me of the life and death struggles Rene had lived through for so long. She talked easily and willingly of Rene Caisse, but of the formula for Essiac, she spoke sparingly and with difficulty. Always, a silent dialog within her seemed to be in progress.

Eventually she admitted to me that Rene had left her a copy of the formula. As gently as possible I began trying to persuade her to trust me with it. Rene had freely given it to this woman, who had guarded it with complete inflexibility for years, and now here was someone else, once again, asking that the formula for Essiac be released.

I realized that for this woman to pass on the formula was an ultimate act of trust, and also her acknowledgment that she had, in some way, finally made her choice and passed on her role in what would happen to Essiac. It was an agonizing time for all concerned as doubts, suspicions and fears came and went and came again.

Our conversations, interrupted by days or weeks of withdrawal and silence by this woman, stretched over almost a year. It was a humbling experience. I learned patience. I learned how to wait.

The break came during one of those difficult periods of hiatus. This was the third or fourth time I had been put on hold, and I was braced for the worst. But when the break came, there was no ceremony. Merely an indistinct message on the tape of my answering machine saying: "Come now."

I flew to the city where she lives, then anxiously waited in my hotel room for several hours. I had a contract drawn up that defined our responsibilities to each other, and to Rene and her formula, in great detail. But none of that turned out to be wanted or necessary.

When I arrived at her home, there was a soft silence for some time. She stirred in her chair and said, "Well, all in God's good time." Then another long silence. Then her eyes, normally a faded blue, were burning. She said, "Gary, there are things better learned by you only when they happen to you." And she handed me a sheet of paper with a list of herbs, typed out, and the instructions for brewing the tea.

She didn't feel like visiting, so I rose and left and returned to Los Angeles, with a formula and my belief that what this woman had told me was true. But I had no proof.

The first thing I did was brew a batch of Essiac for myself. This woman had told me that its preventive powers were awesome; that Rene had drunk the tea every day of her life. And sure enough, within two days I felt fitter than I had felt before. I had been suffering from chronic bronchitis. The bronchitis disappeared. I have been taking the Essiac ever since. It has done me nothing but good.

But that still wouldn't be proof to anyone else. To begin finding that proof, I had only one solid lead: the name of Rene's closest friend, a woman who lived and worked alongside Rene off and on for many years, ever since Rene had cured this woman's mother of cancer in the 1930s.

Rene's friend's name was Mary McPherson and she was a native of northern Ontario. That was all I knew. I finally tracked down her phone number, and when I did it was in—why was I surprised?—Bracebridge.

I called and told her about my conversations with Rene's other friend—though not that I had the formula—and asked if I could meet with Mary in Bracebridge. I could tell that she was suspicious, wary of this stranger, but she agreed to see me.

I flew to Toronto and drove the 170 kilometers to Bracebridge in a blizzard. The snow was so thick and heavy that I could barely see the road in front of me. I don't recall seeing another vehicle for the whole journey.

As I pulled into Bracebridge for the first time, it was hard to believe that this little country town, surrounded by wooded hills and carpeted in snow, had been the center of such controversy for so many decades. Built near the banks of the Muskoka River, it's a lovely town, clean and well-tended, with rows of victorian houses and big front yards. The population is about 9,300—with thousands more who visit in the summer to enjoy the area's water sports and outdoors life.

The rustic buildings on the main street are occupied with shops and stores. There is one movie theater that shows the latest releases. Bracebridge has the appearance of a solid community that is thriving economically.

I drove down Dominion Street, and there was the red brick building, the old British Lion Hotel, where sick people could line up for treatment only if they had a written statement from a doctor stating that they were sure to die—and so were now free to do as they wished.

I knew that here in this town were Rene's records, in Mary's care, long secured in boxes and waiting for someone to come for them once more. I knew that Rene had kept every piece of paper—the diagnoses from doctors, correspondence with Sloan-Kettering, with Premier Hepburn, with her thousands of patients, all the newspaper clippings, the parliamentary testimony. Everything. There were said to be records of everyone she had treated, written in copperplate scrawls on yellowed paper.

I desperately wanted to see it all. I was consumed with the idea that I wanted the whole truth from Mary. I had to "know it all." At the beginning of our first meeting on that bright, crisp, snowy morning, Mary seemed disillusioned and cynical. She had the same guarded manner I had encountered with Rene's other friend. If I had known then what hell Rene and they had lived through for most of their lives, I would have expected her to turn me away at the door.

Mary later told me that there had been so many doctors, lawyers and corporations pursuing the formula that she couldn't take much more of the pressure. She said that she had made a promise to Rene—when Rene was on her death bed—that she would never reveal the formula to anyone, and she said she would never break that promise.

I think that was probably Mary's polite way of saying that if getting the formula was what I had in mind, I might as well forget it, just pack up and go home and leave her alone.

I promised her that I would not ask her to give me the formula, and she seemed to relax a little. As we talked she told me
her own story: At different times in the twenty years or so after
Rene cured Mary's mother of cancer, Mary and her husband Cliff
had each had cancer, and Rene had cured them both with Essiac. With what she'd seen, there was absolutely no doubt in
Mary's mind about the value of Essiac.

After Mary became Rene's best friend, she watched Rene go
through the hell of threatened arrests, promises of millions of
dollars, even death threats from desperate people she had to turn
away for lack of proper documentation—and all because Rene
wanted to cure a deadly disease and not charge for doing it.

We talked for eight hours. I think Mary could see how sincere
my interest was. As she reminisced about Rene, she seemed to
enjoy herself. Her spirits picked up. "She saw it all," Mary said.
"She even had quite a joke with the jailer right across the street
from the clinic. Because she was so big, he used to say, 'Don't
worry, Rene, I'll reenforce the floor. I know you're going to be
with me one of these days.' "

Once when some official showed up with a warrant to arrest
her, Rene went and put her coat on, then asked him what the
charge was. He told her it was giving unauthorized medicine for
cancer. "Rene said, 'Well, if it's an offense in our great land of
Canada to save lives, then I guess I'm guilty and I'm ready to
go.' And the official tore up the warrant and left. They never did
arrest her."

The years of the clinic were Rene's happiest years, Mary said.
"She was a happy person when she had the clinic. She helped a
lot of people and that was always her aim in life: to help people.
A lot of our local doctors thought the world of her. They'd drive
their own patients in their own cars to be treated by Rene. Dr.
Bastedo drove his patients to the clinic. But he got too loud about

it, I guess, and the medical association stepped on him. They told him he couldn't do that any more. What was the man to do, eh? That was his life. So he stopped."

Mary told me a story about Rene when she was a young nurse that sort of summed it all up for me. "She was attending an expectant mother who was going to give birth in her home. The doctors came and made their examination and left. They said they'd be back at a certain time. This was before most people had telephones. They left Rene in charge and before they came back, the mother's labor quickened. Rene saw that the baby was in the wrong position. The baby had to be turned to save the mother's life. So Rene did it.

"Mother and child were resting comfortably when the doctors returned. The doctors were horrified at what she'd done. One of them said, 'Don't you know you could have been sued if things had not turned out well?' Rene said, 'Yes, but if I hadn't done anything, the girl would have died. Then what?' That's just the way Rene was all her life. She used to laugh about that story and say that everything had a funny side. She said the expressions on those doctors faces were priceless."

That night I took Mary to dinner, and I will never forget the look on her face when I recited to her the list of herbs that make up Essiac. She was shocked. Her eyes went the size of silver dollars. For a moment I thought she was going to be outraged.

"*How did you get that?*" she snapped at me.

But then she collected herself and sighed, a deep sigh, as if she were relieved, glad that someone she trusted finally had it without her breaking any promises.

Later that evening she opened up completely, smiled a lot, confirmed the accuracy of the formula, and finally she said: "I don't know why I'm going to do this, but I trust you and I'm going to let you have the documents that no one has seen since Rene gave them to me."

Mary was as good as her word. Over the next few months, I made two more trips to Bracebridge, becoming closer to Mary each time, hearing more of the story, and returning with large suitcases filled with papers.

It took me two weeks just to read all those papers. By the time I was finished reading, I knew I had more research to do, but I was convinced beyond a reasonable doubt that Essiac was effective—at the very least for its pain relief qualities—as a treatment for cancer. I was certain that my initial faith was backed up with cold, hard fact. Reading those papers the first time was, for instance, how I learned of Rene's work with Dr. Charles Brusch.

CHAPTER
ELEVEN

hen I first learned of Rene Caisse's work with Dr. Charles Brusch three decades ago, I thought it would be too good to be true that I might be able to locate him and persuade him to talk with a stranger about his use of a cancer remedy that was not accepted by the American Medical Association—and that might make him a source of controversy.

How wrong I was. The Brusch Medical Center is still in operation and still one of the largest medical clinics in Massachusetts. It has a staff of about 40, most of them specialists, and Dr. Brusch—now in his late 70s—is still involved on a part-time basis.

Dr. Brusch took my first long-distance phone call. When he was actually on the other end of the line and I began to explain who I was and what I wanted to ask him about, I was expecting the same kind of guarded—even fearful—response that Ralph Daigh and Paul Murphy had gotten from the three doctors in Bracebridge.

But the moment I mentioned Rene Caisse, Dr. Brusch reacted with enthusiasm. It was as if I'd said the magic word. He was thrilled that after all these years someone was finally going to tell her story—and present to the public the available information about Essiac.

In my first phone call to him, we talked for an hour and a half. He was happy to reminisce about Rene Caisse. "She was just a young women when she started and she died at 90," he said. "That three-story clinic of hers was jammed. In this little town, she picked up 55,000 signatures. People raised such a fuss that they had to give her permission to treat cancer."

I asked what she was like as a person. "She was a kind, gentle, stocky woman," he said. "She was remarkable, a real saint."

When she arrived in Cambridge, he said, she was still relying primarily on intramuscular injections of Essiac in her treatment. But he worked with her to refine the formula so that the injections would no longer be necessary. They could rely on the oral treatment, merely drinking the tea. "We worked it out," Dr. Brusch said, "and found out that there was too much by injection. You couldn't give it as often as you should, so we changed it over to sticking mostly with the liquid form."

I couldn't believe how outspoken he was on the subject of Essiac. At one point, he said to me without any hesitation in his voice: "I know Essiac has curing potential. It can lessen the condition of the individual, control it, and it can cure it."

As far as Dr. Brusch is concerned, after being involved with Essiac since 1959, that is a well-established matter of fact. That the cancer establishment has ignored Essiac and still does not include it on their list of accepted cancer treatments doesn't change that fact one bit for Dr. Brusch.

I asked him about the tests on mice conducted by Sloan-Kettering in 1959. He remembered them, quoting from their memo that he had received: "Enclosed are test data in two experiments indicating some regressions in 180 sarcoma of mice treated with

Essiac. With these results, we will wish to test enough more that I should ask if you can send more material."

But Sloan-Kettering, Dr. Brusch said, wanted the formula as part of the deal. "They said to her, 'You'd better send us more material and the formula.'"

I asked Dr. Brusch: Why, after all these years and all these cases, have the governments and pharmaceutical corporations and cancer research institutions failed to give Essiac the serious research—and application—it so obviously deserves?

Dr. Brusch was reluctant to draw conclusions. It was the one moment in our 90-minute talk when he hesitated, when I got the feeling that he was holding back. I could tell Dr. Brusch was wrestling with himself as he spoke, his cryptic remarks an attempt to communicate without really saying what he believed.

But even with his best attempt to be polite and avoid criticizing anyone, here is what Dr. Brusch had to say: "The trouble is....all these centers that have gotten a tremendous amount of grants and done tremendous amounts of work, you don't seem to see much difference....These other companies, I can't understand....Sloan-Kettering, they tell you there's a recession in the growth of the carcinoma and keep wanting medicine, well, there's some merit to it.

"You've got to wonder. Is it for mercenary acts? A lot of reports have been written about cancer and all and always a hope of getting close to it, but....we don't get anywhere.

"The medications you can buy now—well, the action of that medication, a lot of it, isn't good....But they're making a great penny on it. Why should they go ahead and—I don't know. It surprises me....But now—I don't know. A lot of people are getting large sums."

But as soon as the conversation returned to the blessing of Essiac, Dr. Brusch's enthusiasm and openness returned. "I know:

the stuff works," he said to me. "It's very inexpensive. You can get a gallon of the stuff for about $40, transportation and all. Just try and get radiation and chemotherapy—and see what it'll cost you.

"And it (Essiac) works! If it doesn't cure them, it will help them. There are no side effects. They're just herbs. There's no addition of preservatives or anything at all. You can continue using your other medications—heart, blood pressure, anything you want. There doesn't seem to be any reaction at all.

"If they (the patients) can go 11 or 12 years when they're told they're going to get two years, and the lymphs clear up and they do fine and gain weight—why don't they give it a try?

"Rene's the one who carried the tradition over from the Indians to us, and it's worked better than all the (other) traditions that have been handed over. It helps. It helps."

Dr. Brusch encouraged me to continue my research and said that whenever I could get to Boston, he would be happy to meet with me and share some of the case histories of people he has treated with Essiac over the years. There were a few, in particular, that he was proud of and who had given him permission to discuss their cases publicly. They, too, wanted to do what they could to help by waiving the confidentiality of their medical records.

Then he mentioned that he included himself in that group. In 1973, Dr. Brusch said, he had had cancer. He had three operations. "I had the Essiac," he said, "and so I was able to take it and I'm still taking it now. And I had a test done a few months ago, and I've been negative." He said he was convinced that Essiac had played an important role in keeping him free of cancer.

Not long after our phone conversation, I called Dr. Brusch and asked if this would be a good time for me to see him in Cambridge. He said yes, and invited me to spend a Saturday afternoon with him at his home. He would have his files ready for me. I think he was as excited about the opportunity to tell his story as I was about the opportunity to hear it.

On a lovely New England autumn day, I drove along the Charles River, then through Harvard Square, which was bustling with activity, as always, and past the colonial homes with their rich history. A plaque in front of one identified it as the home of the poet Longfellow.

A few blocks away, on a quiet, tree-lined street of two-story houses that date from the 19th century was Dr. Brusch's home of the last many years.

Dr. Brusch and his wife, Jane, greeted me at the front door. They're a handsome couple. Jane is probably in her 40s, a warm and gracious woman. Dr. Brusch is distinguished looking, with a full head of gray hair, a warm smile and an alert twinkle in his eyes. On a Saturday afternoon he was wearing a well-tailored dark suit and tie. I smiled at that. I was charmed that the doctor would dress formally to greet someone who'd just arrived from southern California.

But the formality was only in his clothes. I was quickly made to feel at home, a welcome guest. Dr. Brusch gave me a tour of his home and told me a bit of its history. Hanging on the wall in a hallway was a photograph of Jack and Jackie Kennedy with Dr. Brusch.

The dining room table was covered with files and papers that Dr. Brusch had collected from the Medical Center to go over with me. We sat at the table and Dr. Brusch told me a bit of his own history as a doctor. As a practicing MD for more than 50 years, he had long been interested in nature's ways of healing the ill.

Many years ago, as a supplement to standard medical techniques, Dr. Brusch had studied the curative powers of sea kelp and various herbs. He had also studied the value of nutrition in preventing and treating illness.

So he was not inherently hostile in 1959 when he first heard about Rene Caisse's cancer treatment that was based on an herbal formula. After seeing the results on the patients she treated, he knew that Essiac had value. No question about it.

After Rene returned to Bracebridge, Dr. Brusch continued to receive Essiac from her and give it to patients who had no other hope. He found that Essiac worked better on people who hadn't had radiation treatments. It did work on people who'd had radiation. Not as fast and not as well—but it helped.

Then we got into the specific case histories. Knowing that many in the medical establishment—of which Dr. Brusch himself is a respected member—scoff at personal testimonials, no matter how impassioned, and accounts of cures that can be dismissed as anecdotal, Dr. Brusch made it an important point that he wanted to read some of his own carefully documented cases into the record. He had with him the medical papers—the lab reports and such—that supported every statement he made.

There were two cases in particular that he regarded as difficult, if not impossible, to deny.

The first was the 1975 case of a man named Patrick "Sonny" McGrail—who had been mentioned in the *Homemaker's* article in 1977. Dr. Brusch had known him for years. "One day he called me up," Dr. Brusch said, "and he told me, 'I've got something wrong with my stomach.' I said, 'Well, come on over, Sonny.' I found out he had a swelling and a lump in the lower part of the esophagus. I said, 'Sonny, you're going to have to have a little surgical treatment here.'"

McGrail was operated on at New England Baptist Hospital. The surgeon told Dr. Brusch that the diagnosis was esophageal cancer.

After the operation, McGrail was given radiation treatments. Reading from his case file, Dr. Brusch said that McGrail's weight dropped to 109 pounds.

"He called me up and said, 'Will you please see me? I'm going to die. I can't eat. I can't sleep. I'm losing weight. I've got severe pain. I'll be dead in two years.'"

Dr. Brusch told him to come on over. "I had the material all there, the Essiac, the powder and liquid we used to make it up. I kept giving him that, and I loaded him up with the vitamins and nutrition. He improved right along, went up to 125 pounds."

Years later, McGrail's surgeon wrote in his hospital report: "Mr. McGrail is doing well and essentially asymptomatic and looks better than he has over the past couple of years. He saw Dr. Brusch one week ago and everything was fine with his checkup. On examination, head and neck are negative. Lumps are nice and clear. Heart sounds are fine. Abdominal examination is un-remarkable...We are delighted with his progress."

On February 15, 1979, Patrick McGrail wrote to Dr. Brusch: "This is a note to let you know what Essiac has done for me. I was operated on on February 2nd, 1975, for esophageal cancer. After about five weeks my doctor that operated on me put me on radium treatments. I had 11 treatments in 11 days and I lost 12 1/2 pounds. I kept losing weight after that from 156 to 109. Lost my appetite, could not sleep and was very weak.

"Dr. Brusch gave me a bottle of Essiac to see what it would do for me. I was just using it one week when I started to improve and put on weight. I went from 109 to 130 pounds in six months, and the pain eased. That will be two years ago, February 19th.

"I used to take one ounce of it every night before going to bed. Last November the doctor could not get it, so when I stopped taking it, I started losing weight again. No energy. If Dr. Brusch did not give it to me, I would not be alive today. I do hope that it will soon be available for cancer patients."

That note had been written eight years earlier. I asked Dr. Brusch what happened to Patrick McGrail after that. Dr. Brusch pulled out a letter McGrail had written to him just a few months earlier, on May 11, 1987: "I am still being treated by Dr. Brusch for my cancer of 11 years and am doing good. When I was operated on, they said I would not live two years. The Essiac worked wonders."

I asked Dr. Brusch for his own personal comments about the McGrail case. He said simply: "It was the Essiac that does the trick. That's one case."

The second case was much more recent—and even more dramatic. This one involved a man named Ross Nimchick. Along with Nimchick's case file—which contained all the supporting medical records—Dr. Brusch had a written account from Nimchick detailing every step of the way in his own words:

"June 15, 1986. I, Ross Nimchick, came down with a cold and loss of voice. My glands were swollen and I noticed a lump near my left collarbone and in the groin area.

"June 23rd: Appointment with Dr. Clinton. He examined the lump and gave me a prescription and had me go for blood tests.

"June 25th: Blood tests taken at Holyoke Hospital.

"July 7th: Dr. Clinton recommends a biopsy.

"July 21st: Biopsy completed at Holyoke Hospital.

"July 30th: I called Dr. Clinton's office for the biopsy report. Dr. Akers told me I had malignant lymphoma and to contact Dr. Ross.

"July 30th: Stitches taken out from biopsy operation.

"August 6th, '86: Dr. Ross examined me in her office. She measured the nodes, took my height, weight, and had me go for more blood tests. Dr. Ross said I was in the third to fourth stage of lymphoma.

"August 8th: Bone marrow test done in Dr. Ross' office.

"August 18th: CAT scan done at Holyoke Hospital.

"August 22nd: Dr. Ross gave me the results of all the tests. I do not have to return until October 2,'86, unless I feel my condition begin to deteriorate.

"August 28th: I discuss my condition with Dr. Brusch and we go over the vitamins and Mr. Croft's daily food intake program.

"September 3rd: I begin to take my vitamins and start on the food program.

"September 12th: I begin to take Essiac. Two ounces mixed in two ounces of warm water. All water I am drinking is purified by reverse osmosis.

"October 2nd,'86: Dr. Ross examines me and she has a blood test done. I no longer notice any sweating and I feel stronger. I am still on my vitamins, food diet and Essiac.

"December 2nd: Dr. Ross examines me and I have blood tests completed. No treatment needed, although white blood count up to 25.1. Dr. Ross wants me to come in for blood tests January 3.

"End of December,'86: I caught a cold and felt weak. I have increased my vitamin C. The nodes under my armpits have grown slightly and the nodes near my groin have remained the same.

"January 3rd,'87: Went in for blood tests but no exam by Dr. Ross. Dr. Ross informs me over the phone that my white blood count has increased and that next time she may have to start me on medication. I have discontinued my diet and begun to eat pineapple, take vitamin B-6 and I increased my intake of broccoli.

"February 3rd,'87: Dr. Ross examines me and has blood tests done. I have gained two pounds. White blood count has dropped slightly. I have noticed my nodes have decreased in all areas. I have decreased my vitamin C to one gram, my vitamin B-6 to 100 milligrams per day. During February, I noticed my nodes going down about 50%. I feel in good health and I am no longer tired.

"March 2nd, '87: Dr. Ross examines me and has a blood test taken. White blood and red blood count are normal. Dr. Ross said they must have made a mistake and ordered another blood test taken. Same result. Nodes under my left armpit are no longer there. Nodes under my right armpit have gone down 95%. Nodes on both my groins have decreased in size by about 95%. My neck has only one node left, and that is also decreased by about 95%. I feel in excellent health. I am continuing with my vitamins and two ounces of Essiac and two ounces of warm water."

Nimchick's statements are verified by the official hospital records in Dr. Brusch's file. Then Dr. Brusch read a letter he'd received from Nimchick, dated May 30, 1987:

"I just wanted to send you a brief note to say I am feeling great. I am continuing my vitamins, food program and two ounces of Essiac daily. As I look back to last fall of '86, I remember how tired and weak I used to feel. But today I am strong, full of energy and back to my old self prior to having lymphoma.

"I have enclosed a picture taken last December, which shows lumps under my chin. This is the only picture of myself. I have also enclosed my latest report from my blood test of April 27th. My next test is June 22nd, '87, which I will forward to you upon completion.

"In closing, Dr. Brusch, your program with Essiac has returned me to 100% health with no further lymph nodes and a normal life again. I look forward to talking to you soon after my next report. Sincerely, Ross Nimchick."

With cases like that in his files after almost 30 years of personal experience with Essiac, Dr. Brusch is frustrated and unhappy at the lack of attention it has received from medical authorities. But he has no plans to give up his public praise of Essiac.

Why? Because he's convinced that Essiac has too much value to humanity to allow it to disappear. "I don't say it cures everything," Dr. Brusch told me. "But it's the only thing I know so far that can do the work as well as this. That's why I feel so good about this stuff. I know: The stuff works!"

The day after my meeting with Dr. Brusch, I left to visit Bracebridge again. Mary wanted to introduce me to some of the people in town who had known Rene and had their own personal experiences with Essiac. I'll always be grateful for what those good and generous people in Bracebridge shared with me on that trip.

CHAPTER
TWELVE

I n the transcript of the 1939 Royal Cancer Commission hearings is the testimony of a woman named Eliza Veitch. Sworn to oath almost 50 years ago, she told her own story under interrogation by doctors and lawyers.

She'd been operated on in 1935 for cancer of the bladder. "So then I went home and months went on and I began to get worse, gradually going down and getting off my feet. I could not stand on my feet. That was where my pain was. When I would stand I would have this terrible pain."

She went for an examination. The doctor told her that one spot had started to grow again. "So I didn't know what to do. I didn't think there was any use going back. I had my mind made up. I was going to die with it. There is no use going back and being tortured again."

She got worse. She lost weight. She couldn't sleep. When she'd finally given up all hope, she went to Nurse Caisse. That was in May, 1938. "I began to see the neighbors around. My next neighbor was getting cured, and one here and one over there, and I talked to them. People came to see me and told me and this one and that one told me and I thought, 'Well, there is something in it. I'll go in.' I didn't have faith at first."

For eight treatments she didn't notice any change. Then she had a bad reaction. "I thought I was done for sure then but that was the turning point. Then I began to improve and I improved fast."

When she testified, Eliza Veitch said she was at her normal weight of 143 pounds. "I am not saying I am cured yet, but I can tell you in percentage that I am 75% better today. I have cabins on Three Mile Lake, and I look after my cabins and my guests, and last year, I could not hardly walk to the place."

She finished: "I owe my life to Miss Caisse. I would have been dead and in my grave months ago."

Months before my trip to Bracebridge in October, 1987, I had read the hundreds of pages of transcript from those hearings. I'd read Eliza Veitch's testimony and been moved by it. But most of the names of Rene's witnesses had long since faded to the back of my mind. They were voices from the past, people who were all probably dead now, their stories—except for the passages in this obscure transcript—buried with them.

On my second day in town, I went to the Bracebridge City Hall to ask for an interview with the municipal clerk, a man, Mary told me, who dabbled in the history of Bracebridge and knew something about Rene's story. Mary believed he had accumulated some of the documents from Rene's era. When she mentioned him, I thought I heard his name as Ken Beech.

The best I was hoping for was that he might be willing to share his documents and tell me a little bit about what he knew. But knowing the skepticism—even nervousness and paranoia—of the locals who were familiar with Rene Caisse, and guessing that a public official would dodge controversy about her, especially with a stranger who just showed up at his office without an introduction, I was ready to be turned away.

The Bracebridge City Hall is a large, two-story building just down the street from Rene's old clinic. Inside, it is clean and well cared for, with a large open area where a dozen or so men and women keep the tax roles and manage the business of the city.

I waited in a short line until it was my turn. The woman behind the counter seemed surprised to hear that I was from Los Angeles, had no appointment, and wanted to speak to Ken about someone named Rene Caisse. But she said just a moment and walked to the rear of the building and went into an office with a closed door.

A few moments later, she came out and asked if 2:00—right after lunch—would be okay. I think I was as surprised as she was by the answer, and I told her I'd see her then.

When I returned at 2:00, Ken came out immediately to greet me. He looked to be in his 40s, a nice-looking man wearing a well-tailored suit, someone who appeared as though he would be just as comfortable doing the same job in a much larger city. I was impressed and glad that he seemed happy to see me. But I was surprised. His reaction didn't fit my image of how a city official would react to an outsider asking about Rene Caisse. He escorted me into the office and we sat down at a large conference table that sat in front of a desk.

Ken showed none of the reserve I expected to encounter. All I had to say was that I was writing a book about Rene Caisse and that I believed in her work, and he was all smiles and enthusiasm. He opened up instantly. He said he'd already been to his home at lunch and brought back some of the old documents—newspaper stories, the town ordinance granting her use of the hotel for her clinic, and so on—and he was passionate, he said, that the truth be known about Rene Caisse.

"She treated a lot of people," he said. "I can't tell you who was cured or who wasn't cured, but my family had faith in it. I don't know what she had, but she had something that made people feel better. She had something that saved a lot of suffering. There are people using it today."

Ken told me one recent story around town that he'd seen with his own eyes. "A fellow I know had cancer and was on his deathbed, and I know this because I saw him. He was skin and bones and had terminal cancer and he was on his way out. He started taking Essiac and, I kid you not, I saw him a few weeks later and he was driving his car. Now, he still died. He was just too far gone. But when I saw him driving his car, he didn't look bad. He looked sort of full in the face. I couldn't believe it. I just couldn't believe it. But he felt all right. I heard that from his daughter. She told me he really felt good."

Growing up in Bracebridge, Ken said, he heard the stories about Rene Caisse. He wasn't paying much attention at the time. But what he heard did convince him that Rene Caisse's treatment was for real. "She had something," he said. "There are people of high witness for that. It eased their suffering, and by God, what the hell's wrong with that? If you meet my uncle, he'll tell you all that, where he saw people come into her clinic in desperate shape, jaws exposed, just awful stuff, hideous stuff. A few months later, they'd walk away happy and healthy. I could go on for hours."

The whole history, he admitted, had left him with "a hatred for a system that causes this. But I don't know what to do about it. It's pretty hopeless. It boggles my mind."

After we'd been talking about a half hour, I happened to mention the 1939 Cancer Commission hearings. "I think I've read them," Ken said. "I can't say I read every word of them, but I know that it all took place. My grandmother was one of them— Eliza Veitch. She had cancer of the uterus. She was 89 when she died in 1966 or 1967."

Chills went up my spine. Suddenly I understood why this city official was so friendly to a stranger asking questions about Rene Caisse. He was the grandson of the woman whose words I had read and been moved by. I felt a personal connection to Eliza Veitch that I hadn't felt before.

I told Ken that I'd read his grandmother's testimony and hadn't expected to meet someone in her family. "My dad and my uncle can really tell you the first-hand account of the whole thing," he said. "I tell you, I'd love for you to meet them. You can put into words what they can only in their own modest way try to tell you. They're not particularly educated people, but their sincerity will blow you away."

What did Ken personally remember about what his grandmother said about Rene Caisse?

"Well, Rene was like a hero worship to my grandmother, because she knew she was cured. A few of the little things she told me, I can still recall. In every case, she said that after taking it for a certain period of time, there was a sickness, a sort of a weak spell, and my grandmother told me she collapsed out in one of our parks here. My father or my uncle was with her, and they took her right straight back to the clinic. It was after one of her treatments, and Rene Caisse said to her that it was a good sign. That was an indication that something was working, that the treatment was taking effect, and from that time on she started to revive."

What else did his grandmother tell him about Rene?

"Well, there was frustration, a little bit of distrust of the doctors because they fought her so hard. One of the doctors that opposed her so vociferously in those years in the 30s died himself of cancer, and the story goes—I wasn't there to hear it, but my grandmother told me—that he pleaded with Rene to treat him for cancer and she wouldn't do it."

He laughed. "I don't know whether it's true of not. That's the story. But Rene was always very kind, very nice. She had visitors galore. People traveled from all over the country to plead with her to treat their husband or wife. I guess a lot of the cancer treatment is the hope that people feel when they get on the cure. Psychologically, I think that's a factor. But there's no doubt in my mind either that these herbs somehow purify the blood. So if it's not a cure for cancer, then why isn't it a tonic, an herbal tonic, available for $1.00 to everyone in the country?

"I think maybe one of the problems was that it was called a drug. I don't think it's a drug. It's a tonic. You buy vitamins every day in the health food stores and drugstores all across the world. What's wrong with it being used as a tonic? Perhaps that's the approach.

"It's confusing, to say the least, how these things happen. I don't know what the process is where people can get some things on the shelves—here, take this. It's a puzzle. But an herbal recipe, how wrong can it be? What harm can it cause? Why should an association that wants it proven first that it's a cure hold back that kind of relief from people who are dying every year of cancer? What's wrong with making them feel better? I don't understand that.

"My grandmother told me, and I believe this, that Rene Caisse would never have had any problem saving people's lives, saving their suffering, if the local doctors had left her alone. And I have to believe that. My grandmother was a god-fearing woman. The doctors harassed Rene about her business and it was they who took her to task as she was treating people and she wasn't a doctor. God forbid. I expect Rene was taking some of their customers away. If they'd kept their mouths shut...it was awful."

By now, we'd been talking for almost an hour. I was concerned that I might be taking too much time out of Ken's afternoon schedule. When I suggested that perhaps I should let him go, he said, no way. Anybody who came all the way to Bracebridge from Los Angeles to learn about Rene Caisse was welcome to as much of his time as was needed.

He said he had a videotape of a Canadian television show he wanted me to see—the one that aired after the *Homemaker's* article appeared—and he wanted me to meet Mayor Lang. "The mayor, he knew Rene, and he believes, too, that she had something. He knows it helped ease people's suffering and made them feel good, and he'll tell you his own story because he was a personal friend of Rene's, even though he's my age."

Ken took me upstairs to a conference room with a television and went to get the tape. A few minutes after he returned, the mayor walked in.

Jim Lang is a tall, lanky man with the hearty look of an outdoorsman. He was dressed casually and wearing cowboy boots. He gave me a friendly greeting, said he was happy that someone was looking into the story of Rene Caisse, and got to the point as quickly as Ken had: "A fellow who used to be a neighbor of mine, he died a couple of years ago, I guess he was 77 years old. But his mother used to run a boarding house here in town. He didn't marry until his 50s, so he was living at home at the time Rene had her clinic going. He used to tell me of dozens and dozens of people who came and stayed at his mother's boarding house while they took treatments. They were from all over the place, from Timmons and Sault. Ste. Marie and down in the states—just all over the place—and they'd stay there maybe two, three, four months, depending on the length of treatments required.

"He used to tell me of some of them. When they first came in there, you'd wonder how they could even get around, they were in such terrible shape with either tumors exposed on their face or because they were so thin and weak, and he said that when they left his mother's place they were cured, they were just like new persons, you wouldn't recognize them as the same people, when they came and when they left."

The mayor had organized Rene's 90th birthday party, a few months before she died. More than 600 people were there, from all over Canada—and some from the U.S. "A lot of people," the mayor said, "just voluntarily wanted to say something because they had been treated by her for cancer. That sort of thing went on for hours. If you'd been here and heard some of the tributes that were paid by her former patients, it would bring tears to your eyes.

"You know, I often wonder if the treatments that have been performed by research doctors when they test the stuff were done in the same manner that Rene did it. That's the other thing nobody knows, because she certainly had results. She cured people that were given up on by doctors—totally given up on. They said, 'You're going to die and there's nothing we can do about it.' And they went to Rene and 20 years later they were still walking. I know that for a fact because I knew Rene for probably 25 years."

As a young man, Jim Lang had helped Rene out doing odd jobs around her house. "I can remember working in her home in the 50s and 60s. I used to look after all of Rene's stuff. And people were coming into her home for treatment then. Her patient load was down because she had to be careful about what she did, but there were people that she knew and for some reason, she looked after them. They'd come to her house."

I mentioned that the worst thing I'd ever heard about Rene was that she was stubborn. The mayor laughed. "I wouldn't have cast her as being stubborn. She was certainly set in her ways, but I would say more determined than stubborn. She was very determined. If you were having a discussion with Rene, you'd certainly know that you were in an argument before you were finished, and most times you'd probably be convinced that she was right. No, I wouldn't say she was stubborn. She was a very kindly person, very compassionate and very dedicated. She really believed in what she was doing, really believed it. I think if the truth were known, there are probably a good number of treatments that she never got paid for."

After a few more minutes, the mayor said he had to leave. He offered any help he could give, and said: "The stupid part is that we've got nothing to lose (by giving it a try) and everything to gain. But how do we get the right people to listen? It's a shame, you know, every year that goes by, Rene's story is getting buried deeper and deeper. Pretty soon there won't be any of these old people left to tell it."

Ken said that he was going to make certain that I had the opportunity to hear it from his uncle Elmer, Eliza Veitch's son. Ken wanted to make sure that I heard about Essiac from three generations of the same family. "My uncle had personal experience going to Rene Caisse's clinic for months while he took my grandmother in for treatment. To hear his story with the sights he saw and the people he saw come at one stage and leave walking and happy months later is just absolutely phenomenal. He's not going to kid you. These aren't people who are going to lie to you. They're going to tell you the truth. My uncle has a very good memory. He's a great memorizer of poems and stuff like that."

The next day at 10 a.m., I pulled up to park on the street not far from the city hall, and just as I was turning off my engine, I saw an old man struggling up the front steps. He was carrying a cane and he was having difficulty making the short climb to the front door. One leg was completely bowed, as if from severe arthritis. He was slightly hunched over. He was wearing old work clothes. I learned later that he is 75 years old.

A nice-looking, gray-haired woman, dressed up as if on her way to church, had him by one arm and was helping him. I thought: I'll bet that's Ken's uncle Elmer and his aunt Edra, and I was touched that someone who knew Rene so many years ago would take the time and trouble to come to town and climb those stairs to talk to a stranger about her.

I waited until they were through the front door and had enough time to get settled, and then I entered the building. The lady at the front desk told me to go right on in. Once in the office, it turned out I was right. The old man struggling up the stairs was Ken's Uncle Elmer.

But up close and comfortably seated, Elmer appeared different-ly, not a vulnerable, crippled-up old man at all. He had thick, muscular arms and strong hands and a powerful grip. As he greeted me with a big smile, I felt the warmth of his personality. His eyes sparkled, and he was handsome in the craggy way of those old ranchers and woodsmen. He was totally alert, with a quick wit and a booming voice and a loud and hearty laugh that came from deep within.

His wife Edra was a formidable presence in her own right, ob-viously a woman of radiant good health. The thought actually crossed my mind that even though she was in her late 60s, she looked like one of those people who'd never had a sick day in her life.

After a few minutes of getting to know each other, I turned on my tape recorder and asked Elmer to tell me about his mother, Eliza Veitch, and Rene Caisse. In that strong, deep voice, and every once in a while pounding the table for emphasis, Elmer spoke without interruptions or questions for several minutes. Like everyone I met in northern Canada, he has the endearing habit of occasionally punctuating his sentences with an "eh?" Pronounced like a long "A" with a question mark. Before I got out of town, I heard myself starting to do it, too. It's catchy. What follows in the next few pages is a verbatim transcript of Elmer's impassioned opening account. This man can speak for himself:

Elmer Veitch:

This is getting on 50 years ago, and my mother had been diagnosed as having cancer. So she got wise to Miss Caisse's clinic here. Of course, it was going all over in those days, it was quite famous. So every week that was Miss Caisse's wish—that you come every week for treatments. At that time, she administered the treatment by hypodermic needle.

As a result, I took my mother down and we started these treatments every week. I had an old Model A Ford and I was a young fellow in those days. But I'll never regret it—and I'll never forget it either, because some of the sights I saw over here on this corner...horrible. The people were from all over North America. A lot of people from your country came over here.

My mother had the statement saying she had cancer, otherwise they wouldn't allow Miss Caisse to treat her. So every week I brought her down and Miss Caisse told her, "Now sooner or later, and probably sooner, you'll have a reaction with this stuff."

It didn't happen for a couple of weeks, but then it happened right here in the clinic. She sort of went into a kind of a fever and chills, you know, but it didn't last long, not long enough to worry too much about. I took her home. She was all right.

So these treatments went on for, well, as I remember, must have been six months, I guess. She kept taking these treatments and feeling better all the time. So at the end of about six months, Miss Caisse thought she'd had enough, which was probably right.

Now mother lived to be 83. That's 30 years after this happened, eh? Mother lived to be 83 and died a natural death, as natural as anybody would, and the cancer evidently was blocked tight—it never got nowhere.

But yours truly was coming down here every week to this clinic. You'd have to wait a couple of hours to get your turn. It was a big building and the bottom floor was all taken out and seats put all around the big room, and every time I'd come in there, it was on a Saturday, they'd be all sitting around there. Heavens, you thought they'd been there all week.

So having nothing better to do, I went around and I talked to these people. They were very nice people and some of them had half a face, you could see their teeth. Some of them, you could see their ribs. Sights like this haunted me for a long time, you know, and I talked to these people. They talked to me, a good many of them.

The pain they went through was something awful. They'd suffered, and I could see that, you know, but they said since we've been taking Miss Caisse's treatment, thank her and the Lord, we've got no pain. No pain after suffering for months with desperate pains. She stopped the pain.

Now, I don't know, I don't know. Mind you, she couldn't put back flesh that was gone off your ribs or jaws that are gone off your face, and some of them—oh, God, it was horrible, I'll tell you. I can still remember this. It used to haunt me for quite a while.

But that impressed me very much when they told me what they were suffering, and now they had no pain. "Oh, Miss Caisse is an angel," they'd say. I guess she seemed like that to them.

I don't know about a lot of the terminal cases, they probably...but a lot of them got better. Now I couldn't tell you their names. Never did know their names. But I talked to them every week and invariably they all told me the same story: We have no more pain. And they were quite emphatic about that. You can well understand it, too. My mother, oh, she was a great friend of Miss Caisse.

Now about this time there was a neighbor of ours just across the lake from us. His name was Wilson Hammell. He was one of the old-timers in this country here, one of the old pioneers, if you will, and then up towards Bracebridge a little further was another fellow, Burt Rossen. He was born and raised in Muskoka, so I knew these guys all my life, both of them, eh?

They both had trouble and they went to Toronto, to the big hospitals, and they both had cancer of the rectum. They stayed down there for a while and the powers that be told them that they might as well go home. Same thing happened to both of them. They're only going to live a month—you can't possibly live more than a month.

Now those guys were up in years, they were grown, maybe 50 years old or thereabouts. The doctors sent them home, go to your homes, boys, you're only going to live a month, it's impossible for you to live any longer because of what you have, eh?

I remember all this quite vividly. They each came home with the fact that they could only live a month. So, you know, a drowning man will grasp at a straw, and then Miss Caisse was treating 'em, boy. They just went for her like that, eh?

They started out with these needles in the arm, eh? With the Essiac. I can't remember how long they took the treatment, but it was for quite a length of time, maybe six months, eh? Or thereabouts.

I'll tell you what happened. Now this was common knowledge all over. They passed that big black cancer that was in the rectum, both of them, it came away, and those men lived for 35 years after that, both of them, and died a natural death as old men. Now I'll lay this on a stack of Bibles, and I'm not given to lying, I hate anybody that does, but that is actually what happened.

Now, well, everybody around here was completely sold on this deal, eh? So she tried to get the medical profession to recognize her, and I'll have to tell you there was a couple of doctors in this town, they're dead and gone long ago, but they would a killed her if they could of. They said she's only a quack, and the one fella said, I wouldn't take that stuff, I'd die first—and die he did, with cancer.

Now this was the general feeling of the medical profession all over the country. I don't know why. I can't imagine why anybody that could help anybody, God, I don't know why it knocked em, eh? There was people from your country, all over the states. They came to this clinic, and I'll tell you, I witnessed quite a few of them.

They were there every day. I only came on Saturdays, but when they told me about their suffering and the fact that after the treatment started their pain vanished—could you blame them for standing up on their hind legs and screaming about it? I didn't. My mother died, as I say, a natural death, she lived for 30 years after that. She died an old lady in the hospital here in Bracebridge.

That was the end of Elmer's uninterrupted story. When he was finished with what he had to say, I asked him if his mother had gone for surgery or other treatment besides Essiac. "No," he said. "She wouldn't go for the surgery."

Then the conversation wandered for a few minutes. Edra hadn't said a word since I'd turned on the tape recorder. Finally, out of nowhere, she said: "I had cancer, too."

"You did?" I blurted out. I'm sure the surprise showed on my face.

"Three years ago," she said. And Edra, the picture of health, told her own story. She had gone into the hospital in Perry Sound for a simple hysterectomy. But they found a malignant growth on her left ovary. "They took the uterus, they took everything, and they sent it away and found that it was fairly aggressive—that was the term they used. They said I'd have to have further treatment. I said, what does this entail? The surgeon said radiation, and I said, oh, Lord. I felt as if my whole world had fallen apart.

"When he said radiation, I thought, well, Lord, this is the end, or the beginning of the end, and I think I'd better come to terms with it. I had so much experience with the rest of my family, on my mother's side. She had seven sisters and five of them died of cancer.

"I nursed my aunt, my mother's younger sister, for a year. She had cancer of the bone. Her arms broke off here, her legs broke off between her hips. She was just like a rag doll, and there was nothing left of her but a hank of hair and these broken bones. She didn't weigh 35 pounds when she died, and she was only 32 years old.

"It started out a little, wee growth in her left breast no bigger than a peanut, but it was on the breast bone, and she had suffered with a lame hip. She had a little girl who was less than two years old, and after she had that little girl she could hardly walk, you know, for a long, long time, and then she noticed this little lump in her breast, so she went and they did a total mastectomy, just cleaned her right out down to the rib cage, you know.

"It was dreadful, and all the nodes under her arm and everything, and then it came back in her hip, that's where it came first, and her ribs let go from her spine—they were crossed over each over. You never saw such a pathetic and heartbreaking sight in your life, and I will never forget her.

"In those days, they had nothing to treat her. She came to Miss Caisse, but she was so ill she couldn't stand the car ride. So she had to give it up. She was too far gone. Had they got her when they found this little lump, if Miss Caisse had got her then, she would maybe still be living today."

"It was a horrible death. I witnessed it," Elmer said.

"And my mother had cancer—both her ovaries. She had a four pound tumor on one and five or six pounds on the other, and she swelled up like a woman in the last stages of pregnancy. That was in 1948. But at that time, Nurse Caisse's treatment wasn't available."

"You couldn't get it," Elmer said. "No way. They banned the whole works."

"We couldn't get it for mother," Edra said. "It was no longer available."

"Miss Caisse was under pain of imprisonment. She had to quit," Elmer said.

I asked Edra how she felt about that in 1948.

"Oh, I was very bitter about that. I was very angry with the doctors in this town, in particular, for blackballing her the way they did. They really did blackball her. I am not so familiar with it as my husband and my mother-in-law, but my mother-in-law was the closest thing to a saint."

Elmer perked up. "That's why I'm so good!"

We all laughed. I asked Edra how she had felt after her radiation treatments.

"Oh, sick!," she said. "Nauseous, diarrhea, shaky. I would sit and my stomach would go like that—you could see it jumping. It didn't just quiver inside. You could see it jumping with the nerves, you know. Oh, burn, oh! They don't prepare you, you know, for what that radiation is like.

"I had one every morning at 9:30. Well, I was so sick I could hardly get to the hospital. That's the dread I had. After about 17 or 18 treatments, I couldn't even go to the dining room because of the smell of food. I was like someone in the first stages of pregnancy. I couldn't stand the smell of the dining room."

I asked her what kept her going.

"Well, I knew I had 30 treatments to go and I just thought, well, that's one less. Tomorrow I'll have another one and that will be one less, and I took it one day at a time. It was the only hope I had at that point. The last three weeks, I was just too ill to drive the 125 miles to get home and back. I was too ill to even come home.

"In the meantime, he's got this in motion to get me the Essiac. This is what I was looking forward to. I thought if I could just get that, I'm going to get better."

I asked Elmer how he went about getting the Essiac. He explained about getting a doctor to provide a certificate, then getting it cleared through somebody's office in Ottowa, then getting the Resperin Corporation to send the Essiac. A lot of paperwork and red tape, was what it was.

"Then the Resperin Corporation sends it to you, eh?" he said. "For about six months they never charged us a cent. Miss Caisse left a legacy for people, and how much funding I don't know, but we got it for six months and it never cost a penny. Now we pay what for three or four bottles—$40? That's $10 a bottle. You can't measure money against Essiac."

But the first step in the process was written documentation that Edra did have cancer. "I can't really say what kind it was," she said. Some medical term she doesn't recall. "But it was carcinoma."

Weeks had gone by after Elmer wrote the health officials in Ottowa asking for approval to get the Essiac. Nothing happened. So he contacted their member of parliament. "Boy, Elmer rattled their chain," Edra laughed. "I'll tell you, he went right after them." And, she says, the MP's secretary went after Dr. Sproul, the Minister of Health, and before long, they received their Essiac.

Edra had been home from the hospital for about a month.

She was totally beaten. "I would lay awake all night, my nerves were so bad," she said. "It was just like this." She shook her hands, imitating someone who's intensely jittery. "I couldn't sleep. You know, oh, it was dreadful, and then I'd get up and cry at the least little thing. My nerves were just—I was just shot. I hadn't taken the Essiac 10 days until I started to pick up."

She was emphatic about it. "I was so sore from the radiation, you know, my bowels, my bladder, everything. I was so badly burned from the radiation. But I hadn't taken Essiac 10 days when I got up one morning and I said, 'Gosh, I'm hungry for breakfast.' Elmer looked at me, you know, because I hadn't said I was hungry for a long time. But I was really hungry for breakfast. I started to eat again and lose the nausea and the diarrhea and my general well-being—my outlook on life—seemed to improve. I seemed to feel better every day. I've never missed a meal since. I've never had a sick stomach. Mind you, my nerves were hot. I guess—poor father here—I was pretty hard to live with for a while."

She looked over at Elmer and laughed.

"That's when I took to drink," Elmer said.

"I'll tell you," Edra said, "I've been taking it for two and a half years now, and quite truthfully I don't think I'd be here today if it weren't for Essiac. I feel sure. I think this Essiac is my insurance. That's the way I look at it. It's my insurance. I do all my own work. I help Dad whenever I can."

"Dad don't do a hell of a lot, either," Elmer laughed.

"And I'm involved with my church work a lot," Edra went on. "I keep busy. For an old lady of 67, I think I'm doing pretty good. I think I'm very, very lucky, you know. My own doctor has taken blood test and blood test, bone marrow, liver, chest X-rays, bladder sample, you name it, he's taken it, blood sugar—everything is A-1. So praise God, I have a lot to be thankful for.

"I think it was about the 6th of September when I had a checkup. The doctor says, 'You know, you're incredible.' I said, 'No, I'm not. You know what's doing it, don't you?' He says, 'Edra, I really believe it. I'm really beginning to have faith in this medication. You just keep it up.' He's beginning to see that it has done me some good. You see, they're skeptical. They have to be. Whenever there's something new, you're skeptical until it's proven. Aren't you? Well, he sees me on a regular basis and he's beginning to believe that this is really working for me. The last time I was down there, they couldn't find anything. I feel fine."

At this point Edra was finished telling her own story. So I asked Elmer to tell me more about the years of Rene's clinic. What was the mood in the clinic?

"Well, it was subdued, to say the least. But these people knew they were going to get help. Having nothing to do and being a little snoopy, I went around and talked to some of the bad cases, and by God, I'm telling you, there was some god-awful looking sights, to put it mildly, and those people told me that they'd suffered the tortures of hell, for years some of them, eh? That's almost the identical words to what they told me.

"But since they'd been coming here, oh, were they pleased. 'We have no pain anymore, no pain,' they'd say. In big capital letters! So how the hell are you going to dispute something like that? Actual testimony from people with their jaws, their teeth, in sight, and some of their ribs in sight, holes eaten in different places, dirty old cancer, eh?"

I asked how the people felt when the clinic was closed.

"Despair," Edra said instantly.

"Well, there was a lot of ill feeling going around this country at the time," Elmer said. "Damn near everybody you talked to was quite provoked at the medical association. They were so powerful that Miss Caisse was on the verge of being arrested, eh?"

"Heavens, she was an angel of mercy," Edra said.

"People reacted when they closed her down," Elmer said. "But they were more or less powerless. They couldn't battle the powers that be that were against her. It was like beating your head against the wall. But everybody was pretty mad at the time. Those people that were afflicted, they were pretty damn badly provoked to think that nobody else was going to get help, eh?"

We talked for a few minutes about the old days in Bracebridge and some of the people Elmer had known who were helped by Rene's injections. Then I asked Edra how she takes the Essiac today.

"I take one ounce in two ounces of hot water each night, preferably on an empty stomach. Take it on an empty stomach and it goes through all the organs, you know. By itself. It's not mixed in with anything else and you get the full benefit of it. I don't mind taking it. I've rather acquired a taste for it. At first it was kind of, yech. But I hadn't taken it long before I got to like the herbal taste. It's all herbs, that's all it is."

"The Indians knew all the herbs and the value of them," Elmer said. "Today we know nothing about most of them."

"I'd like to see this made available to everyone that needs it," Edra said. "For the medical profession to accept it and dispense it to their patients. If they have the authority to ban it, then they also have the authority to okay it and put it on the market. If they want to charge people $10 a bottle for it—if they've got to make money out of it, fine—but for God's sake give it to people and give them a chance at life! It's not synthetic. It's pure stuff."

"Those Indians, they knew something," Elmer said. "I'll tell you, those herbs can help you. You know if you take the burdock root and black cherry bark, it'll straighten up any skin eruption. It's so damn powerful. You wouldn't believe it."

I'd never heard of that, so I asked Elmer to tell me about it.

"Just peel the black cherry bark off and boil it up and grind up the burdock roots and drink it," he said.

"It's sure bitter," Edra said.

"Well, they're basic elements in a lot of medicines, patent medicines today. It's used in cough medicines to a great extent. But you combine the two—burdock and black cherry bark—and it's the greatest thing there is for any skin eruption. Poison ivy. Shingles."

Edra told the story about one of their daughters. Two years ago she was in tears from the shingles, the pain was so bad. All the doctor could do was prescribe pain pills. "Well, that poor child couldn't sleep for the pain. So Elmer said, 'Well, I'll get something fixed up for her before you come home. I'll get some black cherry bark and some burdock.' Sure enough, she took it for two or three days and the pain was gone and her leg was clearing up."

"Don't doubt it, for Christ sake," Elmer said. "Because it's authentic."

I asked Elmer how he brewed up his homemade herbal shingles cure. "It's very, very simple," he said. "You peel the bark off the black cherry tree, preferably the young trees with the softer and more aromatic bark. Some of those trees get so big that the bark is hard and tough, something like an old man, like myself. So you get the younger trees. Peel the limbs and you end up with a bunch of shavings. The inner part is green, very green. Get about five or six handfuls.

"The burdock blood roots you can get at any health food store. They're cheap as hell, eh? And you put about a handful in the pot and boil it all. Don't hesitate to boil it plenty. It just looks like a very strong tea when it's made, but you taste it, it's great. But you've got to boil it good to get the essence out of the bark, and then like she says, drink a wine glass every day."

"You have to strain it well," Edra said.

At this point Mayor Lang came in to say hello to everyone.

Elmer was calling him "young fella," and teasing him about this and that, and after a while as everyone was starting to leave, I thanked Elmer and Edra for coming to town to talk to me.

"What we've told you is to the best of our ability," Elmer said. "And it's all true. There's no fabrication—none whatsoever. I've witnessed these people that were cured, and I'll tell you, it means something when you witness it yourself. There's one sure way of selling anything. As they say, the proof of the pudding is eating the damn stuff."

CHAPTER
THIRTEEN

T he day after my meeting with Elmer and Edra Veitch, Mary took me to visit her friends, Ted and Iona Hale. Ordinarily they don't talk to people they don't know well about their experience with Essiac. I learned later that they haven't even told the oncologist who treated Iona Hale. But with Mary providing the entree, they had agreed to tell me their story.

On a crisp autumn afternoon, Mary and I left Bracebridge and drove about 20 minutes into the country, through the beautiful Canadian plain country and past small farms. Just outside a village even smaller than Bracebridge, we turned onto a quiet street and parked in front of Ted and Iona's home, next to their big RV.

The Hales came out to greet us. Ted's a muscular man in his 60s, a retired truck driver, with a square jaw and a thinning white head of hair. He's from a clan of pioneer types, one of those guys who's spent his life proudly helping to build the communities of the Canadian northwoods. When we visited, he was recovering from a stroke.

Iona had worked hard taking care of him as he'd gradually gotten better and back on his feet again. She's a trim, nice-looking woman in her 60s, but she looks younger than her years.

We went into their living room, a large, comfortable room with a spectacular view of the countryside. Ted sat in his lounge chair, Iona sat across the room from him, then she nodded to Ted and asked him to just go ahead and tell the story, his own way, in his own words.

Ted had known about Rene Caisse and Essiac ever since he was a young man. He was working with a crew building a highway, for wages of $1.00 a day, and boarding at his sister's. "There was this Mrs. Graham, she used to like you to come in and play cards," Ted said. "She was sick. Dr. Bastedo of Bracebridge said that she had cancer, and if she didn't have an operation right away, she'd die within a couple of months time. She could only be up about an hour a day and she spent most of that hour laying on a couch."

Ted and a friend of his named Tom told her that she should go down and try Nurse Caisse. They talked to her for quite a while trying to convince her. "Finally, she said, 'Well, I can't drive a car. I can't go down there.'

"Tom said, 'You don't need to drive a car. We'll drive you down, and we'll help you in and back to the car and bring you home again and help you into the house.' And she said, 'All right, I'll try it.'

"So we took her down. Her first treatment was around the first of March. We were finishing up the job on the road there about the end of March, and I saw her car go driving down the road. When she went inside again, I ran in and said, 'You know we're going to Bracebridge tonight, right after supper.' And she said, 'You boys don't have to take me down. I can drive myself down.' So she did. She drove herself down, got her treatments by herself. And that fall, she was out playing ball with the rest of us. She was out running around the bases and everything."

Mary smiled in recognition at the story. "I think her name was Elsie Graham," she said.

I asked Ted how long Elsie Graham lived.

"Oh, for years after," he said.

"She lived a long time after that," Mary said. "I don't know how long, but a long time." (A few months after this conversation, I was rummaging through Rene's files and came across a letter written in 1938 by Elsie Graham. "It gives me the greatest of pleasure to write this testimonial in favor of Miss Rene Caisse," she began. Then she said that four doctors had told her she had cancer of the cervix. "I had to keep lying down most of the time & could not work. I could hardly sit in a car to go and get treatments," she wrote. But after four or five treatments by Rene, "I was able to drive my own car." She added: "I feel just fine. I haven't any pain, and as far as I know, I am cured. I have talked with hundreds of her patients at the clinic in Bracebridge who all claim to be helped by her treatments, many claiming to be cured. I feel sure Miss Caisse has got a cure for cancer.")

Ted knew of others from those days when Rene had her clinic, he said, and he mentioned some names: John McNee, Wilson Hammell, Jack Clinton.

But then many years later, in 1977, Iona was diagnosed at Princess Margaret Hospital in Toronto as having cancer of the bowel. The doctors told Ted that Iona was going to die—and soon. "The specialist at Princess Margaret explained to me how sick my wife was. I told him, 'You don't have to explain to me how sick my wife is. I know how sick she is.' He said, 'She can't live only a couple of days. You realize she's not eating anything.' And I said, 'Yes, I know that.' He said, 'She's just starving to death. She's got nothing left. She can't eat because she's full of cancer from the bottom of her stomach to the top.'

"So I said, 'Well, I'd like to know something. I've heard they're trying out this Essiac on a hundred patients here in Toronto, to test and see how well it works. This is the most likely place to have a hundred patients with cancer, so are they testing it in this hospital?'

"He said, 'What do you mean?'

"I said, 'Essiac. Nurse Caisse in Bracebridge, she got this treatment from some lady up north. I'd just like to know where they're testing that.'

"He said, 'What do you call that?'

"I said, 'Essiac. Miss Caisse's treatment for cancer, in Bracebridge.'

"Oh, his face just went livid red. I never seen anybody turn red so quick. He started down the hall swearing something awful. He said, 'That damned Essiac, that damned laetrile in Mexico, it's nothing but a fraud, there's nothing to it. It's nothing but quack medicine. She's just another one of those quacks.'

"I said, 'What do you do for cancer patients here in this place?'

"He said, 'If you're so damned smart, you tell me.'

"I said, 'All you're doing here is keeping cancer in suspension.' And he left and I never saw him again. They gave Iona five radiation treatments and sent her home to die. They said that was all they could do for her. They couldn't do anything for her."

"They just gave me the radium treatments," Iona said, "hoping it would take the pain out of this cancerous stone I had."

I asked them what happened next.

"Well, I came home. You tell him," Iona said to Ted.

Ted said that the ambulance brought Iona home and two or three days later his sister called with the phone number of a doctor in Bracebridge who could help them get in touch with Rene

Caisse. So Ted made an appointment to see the doctor. "I told him what she was like and how she'd had an operation and had a tumor taken out of her stomach, that they'd found she had a type of cancer that would scatter fast, that she wouldn't live long at all.

"After sitting there nearly an hour talking, why he pushed himself back in the chair and said, 'There's no use of you getting Essiac for your wife. It won't help her.' He said, 'I know a girl in north Bracebridge who just died of cancer. Essiac didn't help her one bit.'

"I said, 'Listen, I don't want your advice. I just want to know where I can find Miss Caisse. You kept me sitting here for nearly an hour telling you all about my wife, and then you tell me it won't work. I didn't ask you if it would work. I asked you where Miss Caisse is living. I want to see her.'

"He said, 'Well, I don't believe in it, but I'll take you to another doctor here who does believe. Come on with me.'"

So they went down the hall and Ted was introduced to another doctor. He told Ted that he couldn't put Iona on Essiac until after he'd given her a thorough examination. Those were Miss Caisse's orders. And she had to have a written description of Iona's illness—type of cancer, what the surgery was, everything that had been done.

Ted got their doctor to write up the description, had Iona taken by ambulance for the examination, and the doctor called Rene Caisse and told her that Ted was coming over with a prescription for Essiac.

"I took this prescription up to her front door and gave it to Miss Caisse. She read everything over and said, 'What did you have your wife operated on for?' I said, 'They said she had a tumor of the stomach. They operated and took it out. My wife couldn't eat. She hadn't eaten for a month.' She said, 'Oh, well.'

And she just went and got the bottle of Essiac. She said, 'Now hide this under your clothes. I don't want people to see you taking it out of here. Everybody around's watching me. I'm under threat of spending the last day of my life in jail if I'm caught giving this to anybody.'

"She told me how to give it to Iona: One ounce of the Essiac, measured out in an ounce shot glass, then pour it into another cup, then boil either distilled water or pure spring water—bring it right up to boil—then pour the boiling water in with the Essiac. She said that would cool it down pretty near to where Iona could drink it, and have her drink that the last thing before she's going to sleep at night. Don't have her eat anything for two hours before she takes it. Don't give her even a cup of coffee for two hours after she takes it."

"I couldn't eat anything, anyway," Iona said.

"So on the seventh day about 11:00, I said, 'Iona, you haven't had any pain pills. Should I get you some?' She said, 'No, I don't want the pain pills. I don't need them anymore. I have no pain.' And I said, 'Are you sure?' And she said, 'Yes. I have no pain. I don't want any more pain pills. Just throw them away.' She'd been taking so many of them that the doctor refused to increase her amount."

"The next morning," Iona said, "I woke you up about four o'clock in the morning and said, 'I'm so hungry.'" They both laughed, enjoying their memory of that wonderful moment.

"In the evening," Ted said, "you asked for a small bowl of cornflakes. Then I got her a cup of coffee and she kept it down. Before that, everything she'd eat, it'd just fly right back on her. And then she went to the bathroom all by herself. Then her bowels kept moving freely after that."

"I was down to 75 pounds when I got to where I could get on the scales," Iona said.

I asked her what she had weighed initially.

"A hundred and fifty."

"So about a month after they operated on her," Ted said, "her incision broke open and this cancer stone started to go soft and it drained out. It just kept draining out and draining out."

"All that day," Iona said, "I didn't want to do anything but walk. I just kept walking. I felt as though I wanted to keep going. Then I went to bed and I thought, humm, my stomach feels awful funny tonight, all soft, and I woke up about midnight soaking wet, and there was this *awful* smell. I thought, what's going on here? Finally, that thing moved and it was just the worst stuff you ever saw. It drained out."

"A cup full came out that night," Ted said.

"The doctor came down the next morning," Iona said, "and called it a miracle. They took me back to the hospital and wondered whether they had to open me up again to see if there was any more to drain out of me. But it was all out, I guess."

I asked Iona if she immediately felt better afterward.

"Uh-huh."

And that was ten years ago?

"Uh-huh."

I asked Iona how her personal experience left her feeling about Essiac.

"Great!" she said emphatically. "I'd recommend it to anybody."

I told Iona that I wanted to make certain that I correctly understood the story I'd just heard: When she came home from the hospital, they told her that she still had cancer inside her and that she was, in fact, going to die from it. Correct?

"Yeah."

I asked her if they'd made that fact absolutely clear to her.

"The nurse came in one day and said, 'You know you're going to die, don't you?' I said, 'No, I never even thought about it. I was so burned on anyway, I guess it didn't matter to me, but she often told me I was going to die."

I asked her if she'd had a pathe report when she was diagnosed that came back saying malignancy.

"Yeah," Iona said in barely a whisper. "It was a tumor on the bowel."

Then after the surgery, she had radiation treatments. Correct?

"Just to numb the pain where this lump was," Ted said.

"They said there was nothing more they could do for me," Iona said.

I asked specifically how long they gave her to live when she left the hospital.

"They said about two days," Ted responded.

I asked if they thought there was any hope at all.

"No," Ted said, trying to control his emotions. He was on the verge of tears. "We didn't think there was any hope."

"Nobody else around did either," Iona said. "I went in to see my doctor afterwards and he stood there and looked at me and said, 'Well, here's my miracle woman.' He couldn't believe it. This was in March. It was the first of January when I came home. So I wasn't supposed to be living. The doctor I'd had quite a bit, I spoke to him when I went in and he kept looking at me and looking at me and looking at me all the way to his office. When I went in, I said, 'You didn't speak.' He said, 'I thought I was seeing a ghost. I didn't think I'd ever see you back here again."

Not even realizing it might be a sensitive question, I asked Iona if the doctor had asked her if she'd taken any medicine he wasn't aware of that might have helped her to recover. "No!" she said loudly, rising up slightly out of her chair. It was—far and away—her most emotional reaction of the whole conversation. "And I never told him!"

I was surprised. Surprised that the doctor hadn't been curious enough to ask and surprised that Iona wasn't beaming with pride as she explained to him that she had taken Essiac and passed the cancer out of her system. Why didn't she tell him?

Iona took a moment to ease herself. She thought it over before she answered. "Because I was scared," she said. Then she tensed again: "I thought if I told him I was on Essiac, they might give me a needle, or do something to me that would bring it all back again."

There was real fear in her voice. She'd made up her mind that she wasn't going to tamper with success—and she wasn't going to let anybody else tamper with it, either. "Oh, I wasn't going to tell them," she said. "I got a letter a couple of weeks ago wanting me to go down there for a checkup. I just wrote on the bottom: 'I'm fine.'"

She laughed and Ted laughed. "And I sent it back to them," she said. "No way. I didn't go down for all my checkups."

I asked Iona when she had her last checkup.

"I guess I went down, what? Three times, eh?" she said, looking over at Ted.

"Three times," Ted said. "Last time we went down there I parked the car and ten minutes later, we were getting in and driving away. My wife said, 'No way I'm coming down here.'" They both laughed again.

"The doctor last time," Iona said, "he just looked at my stomach and said, humm, if you keep on in the sun, you're going to be as black as I am.' Because I tan quick. That's all he said to me and I got dressed."

"They kept sending her appointments, though," Ted said.

"Oh, yes, oh, yes," Iona laughed.

I asked Iona if she'd had any prior experience with Essiac.

"Just what I'd heard Ted talking about. Even myself, I couldn't believe in it."

Was there a shadow of doubt in her mind, I asked, that it was Essiac that caused the cancer to pass from her system?

"I wasn't on anything, only the pain pills," she said. "That's all they were giving me. So it had to be the Essiac that brought me back, eh?"

I asked her if she felt as good as she looked.

"Certainly," she said. No hesitation.

Did she ever talk to Rene Caisse?

"I never met her."

If Rene were alive today and Iona could talk to her, what would she say?

"I'd be down on my knees, that's for sure," Iona responded instantly. "I didn't get to meet her because they didn't want too many people going into her house."

Rene's friend Mary agreed. "Rene was pretty scared at that time," Mary said. "Everybody kept threatening her and phoning her. Imagine the pain she must have went through. She had one phone call where they said if she wouldn't tell them the formula, they'd beat it out of her. She said, 'If you do that, you'll never find a thing. Just remember, it's not written down.' Sometimes she'd call me and say, 'What are you doing?' I'd say, 'Nothing that matters, what do you want?' 'Well, I wish you could come up here. I've had a call and there's somebody coming. I don't know who they are.' I'd drop whatever I was doing and go.

"I'd stay in her kitchen, rattling the pans like there might be four or five people out there." Mary laughed, remembering their little trick. "And she'd talk to whoever was there. Afterwards, she'd say, 'I'm ashamed to call you, but I'm scared to death. If it's a person in need and wants to talk to me, I can't turn them away.' She was that kind to people."

The conversation wandered for a few minutes through reminiscences of the treacheries Rene faced from various doctors and researchers—and the ever-present threat of jail. Ted was fighting back tears again, as we talked of how fearful Rene must have been. He mentioned that on his third visit to her, she was so frightened that she initially refused to give him any Essiac.

"She said, 'I'm afraid to give you any. The police are watching my house.' So I said, 'Why be afraid to let me have a bottle to take home?' She said, 'Because if they find that bottle on you, they'll take it off you and that'll be their proof to put me away.'"

But Ted was a desperate man at that point. He promised to hide the bottle in his clothes. Then he promised he'd never tell anybody. Then he finally pulled his German Lugar out of his belt and said he'd use it if necessary. "She said, 'You wouldn't use that.' I said, 'I would so.' She got pretty scared then."

She gave him the bottle and he hid it under his jacket, but nobody stopped him on the way home. As we joked with Ted about his excessive enthusiasm for protecting Rene, he mentioned that he got himself into hot water with her once. She was mad as hell at him. It was over money.

"She wouldn't take any money for a bottle," Ted said. "She wouldn't take anybody's money. She wouldn't let you pay for it. So once when she went into the kitchen to get a bottle, I got out my purse and all I had in it was a $10 bill. I stuck it under a book on the desk and she brought the bottle out and gave it to me.

"When I went for the second bottle, she sat in her chair talking to me for about ten minutes, wanting to know how Iona was and everything, and then she went into the kitchen for the bottle. I got my purse out again and took a $50 bill and slipped it under the book and put the book over it.

"When I went for the third bottle, oh, boy, was she ever mad. Oh! I knocked on the door and she opened it and reached out and grabbed me by the front of the coat and yanked me right into the house. Slammed the door right after me. She said, 'I've got a bone to pick with you.' I said, 'What'd I do wrong? I haven't been talking to anybody.' She said, 'No, you haven't done that. But you left a $50 bill here the last time you were in my house. That's an insult. I don't take money for my Essiac.' She said, 'You've got to take it back.' So she reached down alongside her big chair and got her purse.

"I said, 'Put it away. I won't take it.' She said, 'You've got to take it.' I said, 'No, I don't have to take it. You keep that. The next fellow who comes to the door, maybe he can't afford to pay for a bottle, so take some of that $50 and pay for his.' She tucked it in her purse and put it on the floor and said, 'Well, you put it that way, you can leave anything you like after this.'" We all laughed.

Mary said: "Rene used to say that she'd have been rich if she'd ever got what she'd been promised, cars, money, anything she wanted. But you know something? She got more from the poor people than the rich."

CHAPTER
FOURTEEN

Rene Caisse's family—dozens of nieces and nephews and cousins—is scattered all over Canada and the United States. Some of them barely knew her or what she was doing. Others were close to her. One of her nieces, Valleen Taylor, helped manage the clinic in the 30s.

But even those who were supportive of Rene have tended to play down the family connection, to shy away from publicity of any kind. They saw the crushing pressures Rene lived under, and they haven't been keen on the outside world intruding into their own lives.

Cracking through the walls the family has built around itself over the decades is not an easy task. I was thrilled when one of Rene's close relations who knew her best—and is said by other family members to be extremely knowledgeable about the history of Essiac—agreed to see me after I'd been in town a few days and talking to people who'd lived there all their lives. In his eighties, but healthy and alert, he was polite, even warm, when the conversation was about the natural beauties of the Canadian northwoods and his own past adventures on several different continents.

But he refused to let me turn on my tape recorder and when we began to discuss Rene, he pleaded ignorance and a failed memory—which was clearly not something he suffered from—and quickly shifted into the role of questioner. Why was I there? What was I doing?

We stood in my motel room and fenced like that for about fifteen minutes, and then he was giving me a friendly goodbye and shaking my hand, then walking down the hallway. He hadn't told me anything about Rene, and he hadn't been rude by refusing to see me.

I was impressed. To this day I don't know for sure why he agreed to the meeting. I think he was just curious to meet this stranger who was going around town asking all the questions about Rene. He was willing to spend a few minutes to size up the situation, but he wasn't about ready to open himself up to an outsider, even one sympathetic to Rene. I had the strong feeling that I'd seen more evidence of the paranoia among the people who surrounded her during her life.

But one of her relatives did open up to me. When I contacted him, he said he'd been wanting to tell his story for a long time. He was dying to talk to someone. For years he hadn't shared what he knew even with his own friends. It caused too many problems. He was afraid for his family. He was afraid for his business. He was afraid of the authorities.

Hearing that someone was, after all these years, writing a book about Rene was enough to prompt him to talk. He wanted to talk. Would I be able to guarantee—absolutely guarantee—his anonymity? I said yes, and meant it. He said he couldn't wait to see me. That night he drove to my motel, the Muskoka Riverside Inn in Bracebridge, and spent two hours reminiscing in front of my tape recorder about his relative Rene Caisse and his personal experience with Essiac.

In his own words, here's his story:

I can remember when she ran the clinic. I can remember going in the clinic and what it was like, and I can remember seeing people waiting there. I knew people who were in the clinic.

She wore a nurse's uniform. She was very good, very accommodating to everybody. She was looked highly upon by the whole municipality and the surrounding area. She was always very professional, quite an astute lady in the respect that she could be very hard and she could be very tender, and really quite business-like. Being very heavy and very much out of shape, and in not the best of health, I was amazed at what she accomplished.

One of my aunts had cancer of the breast, I think. I didn't delve into it, but someone had to actually carry her into Rene's clinic. That was back in the 30s, I guess, and apparently the doctors had given up on her. She's still alive today.

After the clinic closed, it was kind of a mystery to me. I knew she had people coming to her house, and it was pretty well all on the QT because it was against the law for her to give this medicine out. So the family never talked about it very much, but we were all very supportive and proud of her. I can remember asking: If this is such an important thing and it was so viable, why wasn't she able to accomplish something legally with it?

I would go and visit her quite often. She really liked to have visits from everybody. She quite openly talked about it, and many times I would ask her: Why is it that you can't do something?

Well, she would explain that she could have sold the formula for money, but the people were going to experiment with it on animals without giving it to human beings, and all of her life she had been experimenting with animals. She had gone to clinics in the states and in Montreal and all over, and as far as she was concerned, she had done all the experimenting that was necessary. All she wanted to do was cure humanity with the thing. But she was astute enough to realize that she wasn't going to give it to just anybody. She didn't want to make a million dollars on it; that wasn't her goal. But she really wanted to make sure it didn't get into the wrong hands. She was dreadfully afraid.

She was afraid that people would use it to their advantage to make a lot of money without helping humanity. That was really what she was afraid of. She was afraid of exploitation. She didn't mind the rich getting hold of it, if they would use it for humanity, but she was afraid that would just use it to make money for themselves.

But really, I never did have it explained to my satisfaction why something couldn't be done to promote this thing and accommodate her needs at the same time. I never could get it through my head. I never did have it explained to this very day why it couldn't have been done.

She felt that the medical association was her mortal enemy, and the Cancer Society was her mortal enemy. The Cancer Society to her was bureaucratic, evil. They were hoodwinking the public, the money wasn't being spent where it should have been spent, and she told me of many instances. Right from the day I met her until the day she died, the medical association and the Cancer Society were her very deep foes.

She felt very strongly that the Cancer Society did not want to find a cure. She said that over and over again. "They do not want to find a cure." There are too many people making too much money out of funds and grants for cancer. She claimed that it was bureaucratic larceny. It was a public fraud to beat all public frauds.

She was in a total state of frustration for most of her later life because her phone would be continuously ringing from people wanting help, and she very seldom turned anybody down. But she was so scared of the Mounties coming and putting her in jail. She would say that over and over again.

I would go for medicine. I would go for a little—the whole family got medicine from her—but she would never let me watch her make the Essiac. She might have let some of the family in, but I don't think so. She made the formula in the evenings by herself—other than Mary helped her.

She would always wrap the bottles in newspaper and she would put it in a brown paper bag and say, "Now you carry that out as though it's Christmas cake or something." I'm sure she did this with everybody. I've gone to her home many times and people would be there. She'd tell me, Oh, that person's from such and such and that person's from Saskatoon, and this person came up from Albuquerque.

People would phone her and beg her for medicine. I don't think she really charged. I really don't. I know that she got a lot of gifts from people. She would point out gifts that she got from somebody she'd cured. If she got money, she didn't get a lot of money. I don't think she asked for money. She might have asked for a donation, but I know that she gave a lot of it away for sure.

Oh, I know she had a hard time getting the herbs. The amazing thing I really can't get through my head is: You take the supposed cures they have for cancer now. A lot of the cures have a very ill-effect on the human body. These herbs never hurt anybody. As a matter of fact, she insisted that they were a tremendous blood purifier.

When I was 18, I quit school and got a job prospecting with a mining company. They'd found uranium. I was out for about six months, I guess, and when I came back, I was out drinking beer with the fellas and I started bringing up blood. They took me to the hospital and I had a duodenal ulcer, a very bad ulcer. The doctor gave me a long list of things that I had to eat and a bunch of milk. He said you keep taking it and by the look of that ulcer, it's going to take about six months to cure.

When I got home, my mother phoned Rene and sent me over. I got a couple of bottles of her Essiac and I took it for about a month. You take it before you go to bed every night, the way she tells you to take it in a glass of warm water, and it's super stuff. Like, you feel good. Mentally it does you a hell of a lot of good. It's like taking a tonic. It's no big deal. It's just a bunch of herbs. I went for a regular X-ray and the ulcer was completely cured. The doctor couldn't figure it out.

There wasn't even a trace of an ulcer. The doctor couldn't believe it. He showed me. I can remember him showing me the two X-rays. The one showed a huge ulcer. The other was clean. But I didn't tell him I'd been taking Essiac. Under oath I couldn't tell him about the Essiac. It was something you never talked about. I never talked to my friends about it. She would go to jail if anyone talked about it. Just to show you how deep it is, the whole family took Essiac, and only one person in the family ever died of cancer. And she was the one who didn't take it.

Rene was death against the knife, and she was death against radium, and she was death against this chemotherapy. She said it was just like water and oil, Essiac and this chemotherapy. People who knew I was related to Rene Caisse would come to me and say, "Listen, how do I get hold of Essiac?"

If I knew them well enough, I'd say, "Well, I'll try and get you a bottle, or two bottles, or whatever." Rene would ask me two or three questions. She'd say, "Is your friend taking chemotherapy? If they're taking chemotherapy, then I don't even want to give it to you. It's just a waste. Have they had surgery? Are they taking radium treatments?"

If they had chemotherapy, she wouldn't give it. If they'd had a knife or radium treatments, she would give them the medicine, but she said once they have the knife, the knife seemed to produce more cancer. When they tried to cut the cancer out, it seemed to inflame the cancer and spread it. That was her theory. The radium—she felt it did more harm than good. She said it killed a lot of cancer, but it also killed a lot of people. But she felt her medicine could still help and could still take away the pain.

She said it would definitely relieve pain. Just that, if it did nothing else, it would relieve the pain, and if it did nothing else, it would purify the blood. She also stated that it was good for the prostate, obviously good for ulcers, and it was just a complete cleansing. That's why I've been taking it on and off all my life.

I can remember in the 50s—or maybe the late 40s—going to visit her quite a bit. She really liked to have us come. She was a heavy woman and found it hard to get around. It was an effort for her to go to the front door, but she baked for everybody, she gave everybody presents for Christmas, even the little kids and the nephews.

She was always cheery. She had a good sense of humor, and she was always strong. I remember one time she broke a hip, and you could tell that she was in great pain, but she would never let on.

She also painted. She was extremely prolific. She would do maybe four or five paintings a week, or more, and she was always giving away her paintings. Like you couldn't go there without getting something because she always wanted to give you something.

My impression was that she was a very strong person, an extremely strong person, not only strong-willed, but strong physically. I was actually surprised that she lasted as long as she did,

and I think the reason was that she had a goal in life. Her goal
was to let the world know about Essiac so that people could get
better by it. If she hadn't had that goal, I think she would have
died years ago.

The worst thing that could be said about Rene was that she
was stubborn. She was a strong person who would say her piece,
and she was able to stand up on her hind heels and talk in front
of an audience. But they could never say that she wasn't fair or
a humanitarian.

I would be safe in saying that anybody who knocked on her
door would be let in, and under duress for Rene. Like anybody
who phoned her long distance and said, "If I come to your door,
can you help me?" I can remember her saying to me that she had
to say no to these people, but I also know that she relented under
pressure from these people, saying, okay, come on.

You know what's funny is that a lot of doctors—and I could
never figure this out—felt that she was helping people. But the
doctors wouldn't admit it. In this little community, as an example,
she knew a couple of doctors who really believed in her. She also
knew quite a few doctors who were dead against it, and she kind
of felt that the doctors who believed in her were scared to say
anything.

She felt that the doctors had a bit of occupational loyalty to
the medical association, and she felt that the medical association
held a wand over these doctors. I know there were doctors who
came to her to get Essiac for patients, and yet they didn't help
her. They didn't help her!

It's kind of a mystery to me, it really is. I know just lately
there are doctors in this community who will give out Essiac. I
have talked to one doctor and told him that I'd heard that he
would give out Essiac if his patients have cancer. He said, "Who
told you that?" I said, "Well, I just heard it, and I happen to be

one of Rene Caisse's relatives. I just want you to know that I admire you for doing it." He said, "Well, you don't have to tell anybody."

She felt that money was the big thing behind it all. She felt that the Cancer Society was a farce. She felt it was a money-making scheme that would be an everlasting money-making scheme as long as a cure for cancer was never found.

As far as the medical association was concerned, she felt that they were so powerful that the doctors daren't breathe a word. It wasn't so much money with the medical association. The doctors were afraid of losing their credibility, losing everything. But she insisted it was strictly money with the Cancer Society.

I think the reason she finally released the formula to Resperin was because they promised her that they would actually use it on human beings. They would give it out to people who actually had cancer. I'm not sure she lived long enough to realize that Resperin wasn't getting very far.

I feel really bad about that. I felt good at first when that article came out in *Homemaker's*. I thought, oh, gee, at last she's going to get recognition and it's going to start going. Now that she's dead and the Resperin Corporation doesn't seem to be doing anything with it and Mary's on her last legs, you know, it doesn't look good at all.

I've often wondered, is this formula just going to evaporate? Is nothing going to happen with it? I feel very bad about it, very sad. We need to be able to give to humanity what's there, what is available right in front of us, and nobody is doing it. The very fact that this thing may die, it's just making me sick. Just making me sick.

My perception is that she helped thousands of people. She used to help all kinds of people that I knew. I'm talking about people who significantly benefited. She always used to say that she only got the people that the doctors gave up on. She never got the people before they were either treated or the doctors gave up on them.

She had a cure for cancer. She has got a cure for cancer. We all knew. A lot of the family were cured. I think even maybe Valleen has been cured. We knew that she could cure cancer, and I think something that we were always afraid of—every single one of us—was the fact that we knew somebody in the family who could cure cancer and that this cancer cure was going to die with Rene. We weren't going to be able to be cured someday in the future. Rene was afraid of that, too. She wanted to make sure that the family was looked after.

The frustration of having the cure, but not being able to talk about it was terrible. Terrible. What can we do to help her? How can we help? Even today, the whole thing has connotations of a mystery type of thing.

Unfortunately, people are forgetting about Rene. She was a legend, especially when she had the clinic, but even in her later years just before she died. But I would say now that most people younger than 60 really aren't aware that something very special was going on here in Bracebridge.

ACQUIRING THE
FORMULA

omething very special *was* going on in Bracebridge all those years. Rene Caisse knew what she was doing. She was helping people with the gift from nature that had been passed to her from a woman who had received it from an Indian medicine man.

As the article in *Homemaker's* concluded: "There's a tragic and shameful irony in the Essiac tale. In the beginning, a simple herbal recipe was freely shared by an Indian who understood that the blessings of the Creator belong to all.

"In the hands of more sophisticated (and allegedly more 'civilized') healers, it was made the focus of an ugly struggle for ownership and power."

I say it's time to go back to the beginning. Let's end the struggle for ownership and power. If you read this and decide that you believe Essiac may have value in your life—or the lives of your loved ones—and you want to be able to brew it for yourself, either as a healthful tonic and blood purifier with preventive powers, or as a treatment for illness, then you should have the freedom of your choice.

I've prepared a simple and straightforward videotape presentation of how to brew Essiac. This is exactly how Rene Caisse did it, the same precise measurements of herbs, the same instructions at every step of the way.

Before I made this tape, I went through the procedure dozens of times—rehearsing the presentation—to make certain that I had answered every possible question that could arise, that I had removed any possible confusion in the mind of someone following these instructions.

The tape is very simple to follow. Using this tape as a guide, anyone—even those with little or no experience in the kitchen— will be able to buy the right herbs in their proper form, brew Essiac and properly store it—and use it.

To be honest, I'm sorry that I feel the necessity to share the formula and the instructions for preparation in the form of a videotape. As I was researching and writing this book, my intention was to include the formula and instructions in written form in the book itself. I don't like the idea of asking anyone to pay for a videotape any more than anyone wants to go to the expense of buying one. Believe me, the purpose of this book was not to sell videotapes.

But the more I thought about just printing the formula and the instructions, the more I thought about my own first experience preparing the Essiac. I had the written information, but when I started to actually brew the tea, I realized that I had questions about whether I was doing each step correctly, with the proper measurements.

I ended up calling my friend. She stayed on the phone talking me through the whole process, and when I was finished, I knew I had done it correctly. My questions were answered. I hadn't made some silly mistake—and remember, even Sloan-Kettering working with only one of the herbs apparently managed to make mistakes in their preparation of it.

My friend told me that one of Rene's deep fears about releasing the formula to any number of friends and acquaintances was that they would make mistakes—and they wouldn't even know it. She couldn't personally train everyone in how to brew Essiac, and if they took written instructions and got them wrong, the whole purpose was defeated.

I'm not going to take that chance. I want people to have the formula, but I also want to make certain that they really do know the proper way to prepare the tea.

As of the time this book is published, that videotape will be available for $79.95 by calling 1-800-537-2472. The tape—compatible with any regular VHS home video machine—will be mailed to you without delay. I know how important this is. I take the responsibility very seriously.